Glossary

α-synuclein: protein that is the main constituent of Lewy bodies

Ballism: high amplitude involuntary movements leading to wild throwing or flailing gestures of the limbs (ballistic movements)

Bradykinesia (akinesia): slowness (absence, delay in initiation) of movement

Chorea: fast, twitchy, unpredictable, involuntary movements, which usually affect the distal limbs and tend to flow from one body part to another

Cogwheel rigidity: a rachet-like resistance or intermittent relaxation, felt during passive movements; used to test limb tone

COMT: catechol-O-methyl transferase; enzyme that metabolizes levodopa and dopamine by 3-O-methylation

DaTSCAN: a diagnostic radiopharmaceutical, comprising radioiodine-labeled ioflupane (^{123}I) in an ethanolic solution, which is administered intravenously; the chemical binds with dopamine transporters in specific areas of the brain and shows up on single-photon emission tomography

Diphasic dyskinesia: involuntary movements that come on with the onset of levodopa response and recur as levodopa wears off

DLB: dementia with Lewy bodies; a progressive dementia, with hallucinations and fluctuating levels of attention

(Drug-induced) dyskinesias: involuntary movements that occur as a result of drug treatment for Parkinson's disease

Festination/festinating gait: characteristic gait of Parkinson's disease with small hurrying steps, often accompanied by difficulty in gait initiation (start hesitation) and sudden 'freezing' of the feet on the ground

Fluorodopa: isotope-labeled form of the neurotransmitter dopa, administered for positron emission tomography

Hyposmia: impaired sense of smell

Lead-pipe rigidity: constant resistance to passive movements; used to test limb tone

Lewy bodies: intracytoplasmic neuronal inclusions found in the substantia nigra and other areas of the central nervous system that are the pathological hallmark of Parkinson's disease

MPTP: 1-methyl-4-phenyl-1,2,3,6-tetrahydropyridine; by-product of pethidine synthesis produced illicitly and causing parkinsonism in drug addicts; now used to create animal models

MSA: multiple system atrophy; neurodegenerative disorder that causes atypical parkinsonism, with various combinations of parkinsonism, autonomic dysfunction (postural hypotension, bowel and bladder problems) and cerebellar ataxia

NMS: non-motor symptoms

'On/off' syndrome: sudden fluctuation from an 'on' state (reversal of parkinsonism, with or without dyskinesia) to an 'off' state (parkinsonism) during levodopa treatment

Parkinsonism: the syndrome comprising rest-tremor, rigidity and bradykinesia

PD: Parkinson's disease

PDNS: Parkinson's disease nurse specialist

Peak-dose dyskinesia: abnormal movements that come on in the middle of levodopa response (usually related to the highest serum level of levodopa)

PET scan: brain image taken by positron emission tomography using radioactively labeled neurotransmitters or ligands

Prodrome: a period in which a set of symptoms may occur before the onset of illness

PSP: progressive supranuclear palsy; neurodegenerative disorder that causes atypical parkinsonism characterized by early falls and abnormal eye movements

Serotonin (5-hydroxytryptamine, 5-HT): neurotransmitter important in maintaining equable mood

SPECT scan: single-photon emission computed tomography used for DaTSCAN analysis (a radiopharmaceutical used for the differential diagnosis of parkinsonian syndromes and essential tremor; *see* DaTSCAN above)

Sphincter electromyography: needle electrode test of the anal sphincter to detect loss of electrical activity in multiple system atrophy

Stereotactic surgery: brain surgery performed through a small hole in the skull (burr or stereotaxy hole) using instruments attached to a stereotactic frame screwed to the skull

Striatum: basal ganglia nuclei comprising the caudate nucleus and putamen

Substantia nigra: black substance in the midbrain containing pigmented dopaminergic neurons

Thalamus: major relay nucleus of the brain with extensive sensory, motor and prefrontal connections, adjacent to the third ventricle

Vestibulo-ocular reflex: the patient is asked to fixate straight ahead, and full eye movements are then demonstrated by moving the head (by flexion, extension and rotation)

Wilson's disease: rare but treatable genetic disorder of copper metabolism that leads to a combination of movement disorders, cognitive and psychiatric disturbances and liver failure

Introduction

Parkinson's disease is one of the most important disabling diseases of later life. It was first described by James Parkinson in 1817 in *An Essay on the Shaking Palsy*. Since then, the disease has become the pathfinder for other neurodegenerative disorders, starting with the discovery of dopamine deficiency within the basal ganglia, which led to the development of the first effective treatment for a progressive neurodegenerative condition.

Dopamine-replacement therapy substantially reduces the motor symptoms of Parkinson's disease in most patients, improving their quality of life and initially appearing to decrease mortality. In recent times, however, the non-motor symptoms of Parkinson's disease – the long-neglected Cinderella of Parkinson's management – have emerged as the key determinant of quality of life and challenge to treatment. Depression, sleep dysfunction, fatigue, pain and anxiety have been identified as some of the key symptoms of the illness, while visual hallucinations, dementia and falls can result in hospitalization and institutionalization. In addition, Parkinson's disease is associated with considerable caregiver stress.

Given the burdens that Parkinson's disease can impose, this book has been designed to provide doctors, nurses and therapists with the latest information in order to improve as much as possible the lives of patients with Parkinson's disease and related disorders. While most books focus on drug therapy, genetic research or treatment for motor symptoms, here we focus on the 'holistic' care of patients.

Since earlier editions there have been many advances in the diagnosis and management of Parkinson's disease and in the care available for individuals with the condition. New genes have been described, and new methods to aid diagnosis such as transcranial ultrasound have been developed. Meanwhile new clinical trials are now being reported with non-motor outcomes.

Developments in therapy such as human-fetal-cell transplantation or gene therapy/stem cell-based therapy continue to be assessed. Meanwhile, the therapeutic armamentarium continues to expand, with improved injection devices for apomorphine, intrajejunal infusion of levodopa and refinement of delivery of deep brain stimulation.

Non-motor symptoms are tied to progression of underlying disease, and studies have tried to address interventions that slow disease progression. Encouraging but inconclusive results have emerged using the monoamine oxidase B (MAOB) inhibitor rasagiline in a delayed-start design, while other trials such as the PROUD study have failed to produce significant results.

Animal models underpin the key developments in understanding pathogenesis and treatment of neurodegenerative conditions, and research continues to seek a true animal model of Parkinson's disease, one that shows progressive neurodegeneration with Lewy body formation and motor as well as non-motor symptoms.

An overwhelming body of evidence and patient testimony underlines the importance of non-motor symptoms, the need for multidisciplinary care and the use of tools that empower patients. Guidelines highlighting the important role of multidisciplinary care have been published, while the focus of research has shifted from a bias towards motor symptoms to non-motor symptoms, with the publication of specific tools to assess and flag these important problems.

In the updating of this fourth edition of *Fast Facts: Parkinson's Disease*, we have sought to address all of these aspects. Importantly, we have consulted with patients and sought to reflect their perspectives throughout. People with Parkinson's disease require multidisciplinary professional care. When they ask questions they must feel assured that the answers are well informed and correct. This truly useful and unique resource is therefore essential reading for the whole team.

Acknowledgments

We would like to thank Dr Chris Clough and Professor Kapil Sethi for their contribution to past editions of this title. Also, for their thoughtful input into this new edition, Parkinson's UK, The Cure Parkinson's Trust, The Community for Research Involvement and Support for People with Parkinson's (CRISP) group, Joyce Lykke Schmidt, Lisa Klingelhoefer, Lauren Perkins, Louise Ebenezer and Anthony Duffy.

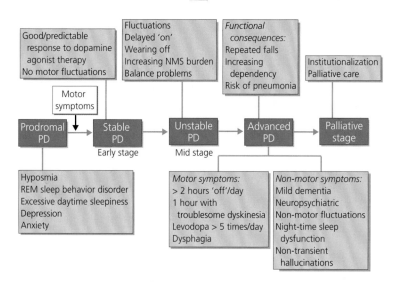

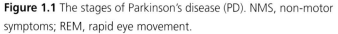

Figure 1.1 The stages of Parkinson's disease (PD). NMS, non-motor symptoms; REM, rapid eye movement.

Prodromal Parkinson's disease

The Parkinson's journey may begin long before diagnosis, as Parkinson's disease is now recognized to have a prodromal period dominated by a number of non-motor symptoms. These are late-onset hyposmia or anosmia, rapid eye movement (REM) behavior disorder, episodes of major depression or anxiety, and excessive daytime sleepiness. This prodromal period could last up to 20 years before awareness of the motor symptoms that mark the initial or 'stable' period of the condition. Those who have the non-motor prodrome will have had unexplained symptoms for years, while those with a dominant motor presentation may have had symptoms for only a few months.

Diagnosis

For the clinician, diagnosis is based on clinical presentation, as there is still no reliable diagnostic test. While the cardinal motor symptoms

9

and signs of rest tremor, akinesia and rigidity remain the mainstay of diagnosis, the prodrome of non-motor symptoms described above develops in the majority of patients. At least half of all patients experience mood disturbance with anxiety or depression at some stage of the illness, including in the prodromal phase.

> *"It was almost a relief to be diagnosed with PD. Up until then I had been told I was suffering from work-related stress and anxiety. I thought it was PD before it was diagnosed so it did not come as a shock. In some ways it was good to know that there was a physical reason why I could no longer cope at work."*

Delivering the diagnosis. Care must be taken in how the diagnosis is delivered. Patients are often fearful and may come to the clinician with preconceptions based on information overload from the internet, or a limited understanding or experience of the disease from the media or a relative. It is best to break the news of a patient's diagnosis in the presence of their spouse, partner or other family members.

Often, little information is retained from that first consultation and it is necessary to meet again within 2–3 weeks when the patient's initial shock has subsided.

> *"When my husband finally emerged from that consultation, his face was completely expressionless. He rushed past me, down the stairs, over the parking lot and I ran after him ... there he sat with his head in his hands and tears streaming down his face."*

> *"Please remember the effects of the diagnosis on the spouse as well. The shock can be just as bad for them and the long-term effects can be severe, as they have to support their loved one as they watch what they go through."*

Satisfaction with the initial explanation of the diagnosis has been shown to continue to have an independent effect on quality of life even much later in the illness. Reinforcing the diagnosis and the steps made to confirm it should be followed by provision of information and advice. A sense of optimism must be encouraged.

• The disease is only slowly progressive.
• There are many effective symptomatic therapies that can help maintain quality of life for the majority of the illness.
• Major research efforts are in force to discover additional therapies and, of course, a cure.

Regardless of the stage of the disease, non-motor symptoms, in particular depression or mood disturbance, dominate as the predictor of quality of life. It is useful to guide the patient to a viewpoint whereby the focus is maintaining quality of life, rather than defining themselves by their Parkinson's disease, and it is therefore important to address both non-motor and motor symptoms, and to treat both social and motor disability.

Early-stage stable Parkinson's disease

Many patients who have already been diagnosed will have read on the internet, or will even have been told by another clinician, that treatment is only effective for 5 years. Inevitably, they will conclude that they should delay treatment in order to obtain its benefits when really needed. It is important to recognize the patient who has this misconception in order to unequivocally dispel it.

Patients who may not have fully accepted the diagnosis may be fearful of treatment. It is important to acknowledge this, and to help the patient deal with their fear and denial. Evidence shows that quality of life deteriorates in those who delay treatment compared with those who start it straight away. In early Parkinson's disease, motor and non-motor symptoms can be controlled in a stable fashion with relatively simple medication regimens.

Initial therapy. No treatment has been shown to unequivocally slow disease progression, although the results of the ADAGIO study of early treatment with rasagiline are compatible with a disease-

11

modifying effect (see pages 90–1). Rasagiline, dopamine agonists and levodopa are all reasonable choices for initial therapy, each with their relative benefits and potential side effects. There is also increasing evidence for the benefits of exercise or physical therapy, even in early or mild Parkinson's disease.

> *"Things that can help ... stay active, both physically and mentally. Talk, sing, go for long walks, do crosswords or sudoku, watch your diet. Above all, remember to smile! Children, especially, do not know how to react if grandpa never smiles at them. It can be done with practice!"*

Mid-stage unstable Parkinson's disease

In most patients, the early stable period of disease eventually develops into an unstable mid stage, which remains poorly defined. It is usually the start of unpredictable responses to oral dopaminergic drugs, with the benefit of short-acting drugs (usually levodopa) wearing off from one dose to the next, necessitating incremental treatment over a period of months or years. Patients experience some balance issues, fear of falling, early morning off periods and dyskinesias.

Initially, this may only occur after overnight deprivation (early morning akinesia) but eventually the wearing off symptoms will occur between daytime doses as well. Patients can experience a return of any of their motor symptoms (tremor, slowness or stiffness).

Common non-motor fluctuations are off-period anxiety, depression or fogginess of thought. Around the same time, although not necessarily linked, many patients experience involuntary movements in response to their dopaminergic therapy (dyskinesias). This is most common at peak doses but is also frequently a beginning-of-dose and/or end-of-dose phenomenon (e.g. early morning foot dystonia, diphasic dyskinesias).

The multidisciplinary team has a crucial role during this period to reassure the patient and carer, re-evaluate motor and non-motor symptoms and ensure that appropriate appointments for physiotherapy and speech and language therapy are made. For some patients, assessment of their ability to drive and/or to continue working in a stressful job etc. also needs to be considered at this stage.

Unpredictable fluctuations. Initially, motor and non-motor fluctuations tend to be predictable and can often be managed successfully by adjusting oral medications to try to achieve more constant levels of dopaminergic stimulation. However, over a period of years, the fluctuations can become increasingly unpredictable.

Unpredictable motor fluctuations are especially disabling, as patients begin to lose confidence in their ability to go out, resulting in increasing social isolation. Unpredictable motor fluctuations are probably linked to unpredictable and often delayed gastric emptying. This results in unpredictable gut absorption of levodopa, which is only absorbed after passage through the stomach into the small intestine. Although patients can still improve with adjustments to their oral medications, this usually only offers limited control.

> *"The Parkinson's Disease Nurse Specialist can play a major role in maintaining quality of life by helping both the patient and carer understand the timing and dosing of medication in relation to the digestive system. Also, being actively involved in optimizing dopaminergic treatment can help to reduce carer stress."*

Advanced therapy. It is at this stage that treatment with an advanced therapy (apomorphine, levodopa–carbidopa intestinal gel or deep brain stimulation) should be considered. These bypass or eliminate the need for reliable gastric emptying.

Advanced Parkinson's disease

Mid-stage Parkinson's disease leads on to an advanced stage of disease associated with a range of motor and non-motor functional consequences. In some patients, the final stages of Parkinson's disease may involve the development and delivery of palliative care.

As Parkinson's disease progresses, some of the motor symptoms that once were levodopa responsive (e.g. fine motor skills, postural

13

reflexes, freezing of gait) become only partially or occasionally levodopa responsive. This can result in increasing motor disability and complications such as frequent falls. Cognitive impairment or dementia can develop, as well as psychiatric manifestations such as hallucinations without insight, or even psychosis.

Fortunately, it is increasingly recognized that the major risk factor for these complications is age, rather than simply the duration of Parkinson's disease. Patients should be reassured that regardless of when their Parkinson's disease developed (fifth, sixth or seventh decade), these complications do not tend to occur until patients enter their eighth or ninth decade, so not all patients will reach this stage of Parkinson's disease.

Specialist care. Treatment of this stage of the disease remains the greatest challenge in the modern era. Treatments that can provide some maintenance or enhancement of quality of life are available, but the therapeutic options for many symptoms are limited. It is important that people with Parkinson's disease continue to experience care from a specialist, who can best help navigate the route between over- and under-treatment.

Patient education. Patients should be encouraged to learn about their condition. Patient support groups can help with this (see Useful resources, pages 161–3). Carer stress is common, and must be recognized and managed. Gentle but accurate explanation of what is happening is important so that both patients and carers maintain some sense of control.

"I felt that becoming involved in a patient support group, and wanting to know more, reassured my family who give me enouragement and support on this 'journey'."

Key points – the Parkinson's journey

- Patients may experience unexplained symptoms for years before diagnosis: prodromal non-motor symptoms, such as impaired sense of smell, constipation and rapid eye movement sleep behavior disorder, develop in the majority of patients.
- Care must be taken in delivering the diagnosis. It is best if the patient is accompanied by a spouse, partner or other family member, and information may need to be repeated 2–3 weeks later when the shock has subsided.
- It is important to address both non-motor and motor symptoms, and to treat both social and motor disability.
- Early treatment is important; quality of life deteriorates in those who delay treatment.
- Maintaining an active lifetyle, both physically and mentally, is important.
- All patients will eventually experience motor (and often non-motor) fluctuations, with a 'wearing off' of the benefit of their initial medication.
- Patients should be reassured that the increasing motor disability and complications of late-stage Parkinson's disease do not tend to occur until the eighth or ninth decade of life; not all patients will reach this stage of Parkinson's disease.

Key references

Clarke C. Medical management of Parkinson's disease. *J Neurol Neurosurg Psychiatry* 2002;72 Suppl 1:I22–7.

Hayes MW, Fung VS, Kimber TE, O'Sullivan JD. Current concepts in the management of Parkinson's disease. *Med J Aust* 2010;192:14–19.

Rascol O, Fitzer-Atlas CJ, Hauser R et al. A double-blind, delayed-start trial of rasagaline in Parkinson's disease (the ADAGIO study): prespecified and post-hoc analyses of the need for additional therapies, changes in UPDRS scores, and non-motor outcomes. *Lancet Neurol* 2011;10:415–23.

Epidemiology

Parkinson's disease is one of the most common neurodegenerative diseases, but estimating its incidence and prevalence is problematic as there is no 'in-life' marker for idiopathic Parkinson's disease; the diagnosis can only be made with certainty if Lewy bodies (intracytoplasmic aggregations of misfolded protein in the brain) are found in the substantia nigra and other brain regions after death (see pages 19–21). Case ascertainment in community studies is difficult, and often other parkinsonian syndromes may be included.

Incidence and prevalence. 'Incidence' is the number of new cases in a specified time frame, and is not modified by factors affecting survival. Estimates of the annual incidence of Parkinson's disease are in the range of 4–20 per 100 000 individuals. The variability is accounted for by differences in the populations studied and by inclusion or exclusion of other clinical entities, such as essential tremor.

'Prevalence' is the total number of cases in a given population at one time. A widely accepted approximate figure for the prevalence of Parkinson's disease is 200 per 100 000 individuals. In the USA, between 750 000 and 1.5 million people are estimated to have the disease. In the UK, there are approximately 120 000–130 000 diagnosed cases but many more affected individuals may remain undiagnosed; prevalence is predicted to rise to around 160 000 in the next 8 years, largely as a result of increased life expectancy. Worldwide figures are expected to double by 2030, rising from 4.1 million in 2005 to 8.7 million by 2030.

Age, sex and ethnicity. Both the incidence and prevalence of Parkinson's disease increase with age, and the prevalence may be as high as 1 in 50 for patients over the age of 80 years. The disease is estimated to affect 1% of 70-year-olds, but is also seen in younger people, with 10% of cases occurring before the age of 50.

Men are 1.5 times more likely than women to develop the condition.

Parkinson's disease has been found in all the ethnic populations studied; however, sporadic reports suggest that patterns of parkinsonism may differ between different ethnic groups. While well-conducted epidemiological studies in black and some Asian populations (such as south Asia) are still lacking, hospital-based studies and some community studies (e.g. the Copiah County study) have suggested that Parkinson's disease is less common in black populations than other ethnic groups. However, this is not widely accepted.

Mortality. In 1967, Hoehn and Yahr published the first mortality study of Parkinson's disease in the pre-levodopa era. They found that up to 61% of patients were severely disabled or dead after 5–9 years of follow-up, which increased to more than 80% in those followed up for more than 10 years. Overall, in this early study, mortality was three times that expected in the general population. Of more than 20 reports on Parkinson's disease and mortality, 11 reported mortality increases of 1.5–twofold, while the others reported increases greater than twofold.

Several researchers have suggested that disability and mortality in Parkinson's disease show a sex difference, with significantly greater mortality in women. However, there are other studies suggesting a poorer prognosis in men. Berger reported relative risks of death of 3.1 for men and 1.8 for women with the disease, although these figures are much higher than those reported in other studies. A study by Japanese investigators suggested a mean age at death of 71.9 years in men and 74.2 years for women. In Japan, female patients appear to lose approximately 7 years of longevity compared with men once Parkinson's disease is diagnosed.

Although some would say that the life expectancy of patients with Parkinson's disease appears to have been prolonged, their lifespan is still probably less than that of the general population, as indicated in the Japanese study. The cause is complex. Improved survival is thought to be a result of the introduction of effective symptomatic therapy such as levodopa, while decreased or delayed mortality from comorbidity may partly account for the decreased mortality in younger people. Studies have suggested that relative survival for people with Parkinson's disease diagnosed before the age of 60 is similar to that for the general population, but for those who are older at diagnosis relative survival is less than expected.

In general, before the use of levodopa the relative risk of death with Parkinson's disease was about 3.0. The 15-year follow-up study of the Sydney cohort by Hely and colleagues, published in 2005, indicated that modern treatment had reduced this risk to 1.86. However, reassessment of this cohort by the same researchers at 20 years reported a revised risk similar to the pre-levodopa era of 3.1. So the longer people live with Parkinson's disease, the higher the mortality rate. It is also important to note that the surviving patients have significant problems: 83% have dementia.

The confusion regarding mortality in Parkinson's disease may be partly because the disease itself is not a primary or direct cause of death. In the USA, the average annual age-adjusted Parkinson's disease mortality between 1962 and 1984 was estimated as 2 deaths per 100 000 for white men and 1 death per 100 000 for non-white men, 1 death per 100 000 for white women and less than 1 death per 100 000 for non-white women. Mortality increased for persons aged 75 years and older, but declined for those younger than 70 years. Overall, published evidence suggests that mortality for Parkinson's disease increases in the older age groups but decreases for younger ages. The cause of death in Parkinson's disease is most commonly a secondary comorbid disorder. A Japanese study showed that the most common cause of death for all patients, regardless of age, was pneumonia.

Economic burden. Studies suggest that Parkinson's disease adversely affects the health-related quality of life of patients and imposes a significant economic burden on society comparable with that of other chronic conditions such as congestive heart failure, diabetes and stroke. Although it is difficult to measure the specific economic cost of Parkinson's disease, in the UK the annual direct cost of managing patients with Parkinson's disease at home is estimated at around £4189; the cost rises to £19 338 for full-time institutionalization.

Furthermore, the total direct cost of Parkinson's disease in patients in 'good health' is three times lower than for those in 'poor health'. These figures do not take into account hidden indirect costs such as loss of income from premature retirement, for both the patient and carer.

Pathology

The main pathological feature of Parkinson's disease is the degeneration of neuromelanin-containing neurons in the pars compacta of the substantia nigra (Figure 2.1). Examination with the naked eye reveals pallor of this area, which is confirmed microscopically by a marked decrease in the number of neuromelanin-containing cells and the presence of Lewy bodies in the remaining nigral neurons.

Degeneration of pigmented neurons in the brainstem is not limited to the nigra but extends to the locus ceruleus and the dorsal motor nucleus of the vagus.

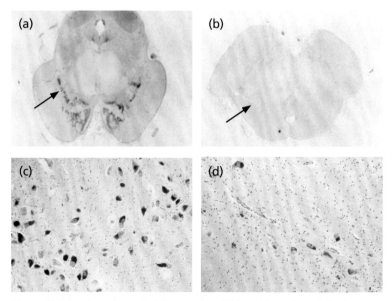

Figure 2.1 Sections through (a) normal and (b) parkinsonian midbrain showing a characteristic loss of pigmentation in the substantia nigra (arrowed). Micrographs of the substantia nigra reveal (c) normal pigmented neurons in a normal brain and (d) the loss of pigmented neurons in a brain affected by Parkinson's disease.

Lewy bodies are intracytoplasmic eosinophilic inclusions, which are found in several areas of the brain but typically in the neurons of the substantia nigra (Figure 2.2). They are a pathological hallmark of idiopathic Parkinson's disease and are also found in other neurodegenerative diseases, such as dementia with Lewy bodies and Alzheimer's disease. Electron microscopy reveals that Lewy bodies are composed of filamentous material arranged in circular and linear profiles, sometimes radiating from an electron-dense core. Lewy bodies stain positively for ubiquitin and α-synuclein.

Neurites are tiny projections growing from the neurons, and inclusions positive for α-synuclein within these projections are referred to as Lewy neurites. Lewy neurites are more widespread than well-delineated Lewy bodies. This has led to a re-examination of how Parkinson's disease pathology evolves.

After examining a large number of brains, both clinically normal and with Parkinson's disease, Braak et al. suggested that stage 1 of the disease begins at induction sites in the olfactory system and the dorsal vagal nucleus, with degeneration of the olfactory bulb and the anterior olfactory nucleus. This presents clinically as olfactory dysfunction. Stage 2 reflects progression of the pathological process to the nuclei of the caudal brainstem (the locus ceruleus and other nuclei). The lower

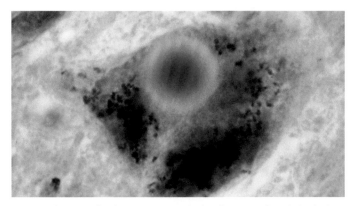

Figure 2.2 The Lewy body is a concentric, hyaline cytoplasmic inclusion with a clear halo around a dense central region, as seen here within a pigmented neuron. The presence of these Lewy bodies is characteristic of Parkinson's disease.

brainstem nuclei are key areas mediating a myriad of non-motor symptoms such as sleep homeostasis, depression, fatigue, cognitive problems, pain, constipation and a reduction in central autonomic vagal control. Several of these symptoms are now recognized as possible prodromal features of Parkinson's disease. However, clinical Parkinson's disease tends to be recognized by healthcare professionals only when the condition reaches stage 3, which involves the substantia nigra. Stages 4 to 6 represent further pathological progression to the cortex (Figure 2.3).

It must be emphasized that the Braak classification is controversial as it relies on the concept of Lewy-neurite formation alone and not on neuronal degeneration. In addition, other researchers have found that this pattern of pathological progression is not seen in all brains. For instance, it is now recognized that some people with Parkinson's disease express cognitive and other symptoms such as apathy at the onset of the motor condition, which does not tie in with Braak's hypothesis.

A mouse model suggesting a gastrointestinal route for the pathogenesis of Parkinson's disease has also been reported. There is now growing evidence for an upper gastrointestinal origin of Lewy body pathology; animal model studies have shown that such a process can spread via the vagal route to the dorsal nucleus of the vagus, which corresponds to Braak stages 1 and 2.

As Braak's six-stage theory and other clinical studies indicate, Parkinson's disease is a very complex disorder and the motor manifestations required to make a diagnosis are just the tip of the iceberg.

Neuronal degeneration. The cause of neuronal degeneration in Parkinson's disease is unknown. The susceptible neurons are located in astroglial-poor regions such as the ventral tier. Glia may offer neuroprotection by providing neurotrophic factors that prevent cell death. Several hypotheses for neuronal degeneration have been proposed, including:

- oxidative stress, induced by dopamine metabolism or other factors
- defective mitochondrial energy metabolism
- excitotoxin- and xenobiotic-related cell death
- programmed cell death (apoptosis)
- protein misfolding, including the prion hypothesis.

(a)

(b)

(c)

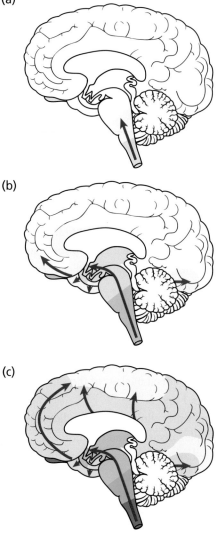

Figure 2.3 The pathological process in Parkinson's disease. Braak's six-stage classification relates pathology to disease phase: (a) stages 1 and 2, which are prodromal; (b) stages 3 and 4, which manifest as clinical disease; and (c) stages 5 and 6, which are associated with cognitive impairment. Adapted from Braak et al. 2004.

Oxidative stress. Free radicals, produced by dopamine metabolism, may result in the production of hydrogen peroxide and very reactive hydroxyl radicals. These can injure the phospholipid layer of the cell membrane and induce apoptosis, and can also damage other molecules, such as DNA and proteins. Free radicals are scavenged by enzyme systems, including glutathione and superoxide dismutase.

Pathological studies have shown reduced glutathione levels in patients who died from Parkinson's disease, suggesting excessive utilization of glutathione by free radicals. Although there is some evidence that cell injury related to free radicals is implicated in Parkinson's disease, this is not certain. A free-radical scavenger, such as selegiline, has no definite effect on disease progression.

The substantia nigra contains high levels of iron. Free iron can induce decomposition of lipid and peroxide, and formation of hydroxyl radicals. Iron levels are increased in brains affected by Parkinson's disease, as well as in other neurodegenerative disorders. This may, however, be secondary to neurodegeneration.

Defective mitochondrial energy metabolism. The study of the toxin 1-methyl-4-phenyl-1,2,3,6-tetrahydropyridine (MPTP) has afforded an insight into defects in mitochondrial energy metabolism in Parkinson's disease (Figure 2.4). Originally, MPP⁺ (the active by-product of MPTP) was thought to damage dopaminergic neurons by production of free radicals; subsequently, it has been found that MPP⁺ inhibits complex 1

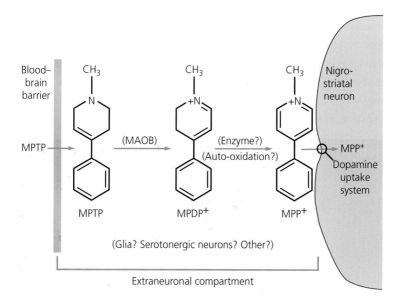

Figure 2.4 The metabolic fate of 1-methyl-4-phenyl-1,2,3,6-tetrahydropyridine (MPTP). MAOB, monoamine oxidase B.

(reduced nicotinamide adenine dinucleotide [NADH], coenzyme Q 1 reductase) in the mitochondrial energy cycle. The resulting paralysis of energy production may account for the degeneration of dopaminergic neurons in MPTP primate models
as well as in humans developing symptoms resembling those of Parkinson's disease with MPTP. Many studies have found complex 1 defects in patients with Parkinson's disease. However, it should be noted that parkinsonism is rare in people with mitochondrial disorders.

Excitotoxin/xenobiotic metabolism. Defects in the enzymes that break down endogenous and exogenous chemicals (such as excitotoxins and xenobiotics, respectively) are seen in patients with Parkinson's disease. Several environmental toxins, including organochloropesticides, may be toxic to mitochondria. It is possible that these chemicals are not metabolized effectively in such patients, which may account for susceptibility to the condition.

Nigral cell loss. There is gradual loss of pigmented neurons in the substantia nigra with age. It is estimated that 70–80% of nigral neurons are lost before clinical symptoms of Parkinson's disease become apparent. However, on 6-fluorodopa positron emission tomography (PET) scans, the threshold appears to occur when approximately 50% of fluorodopa uptake is lost. This difference may reflect overactivity of the remaining nigral neurons in an effort to maintain nigrostriatal dopamine transmission (Figure 2.5).

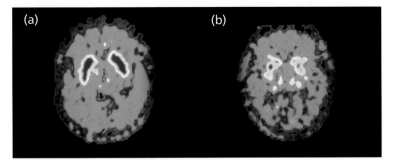

Figure 2.5 Positron emission tomography scans showing uptake of radiolabeled fluorodopa by the basal ganglia in (a) a normal brain and (b) the brain of a patient with Parkinson's disease, in which the uptake is reduced.

Protein misfolding – the prion hypothesis. In several contemporary postmortem case reports, the brain tissues of patients with Parkinson's disease who had received embryonic cell transplants were shown to have developed Lewy body inclusions in previously healthy transplant cells. These sporadic observations have sparked research to determine how normal healthy cells may acquire Parkinson's disease. It has been suggested that a prion-disorder-type condition may cause the spread of the disease. Prion expression is based on propagation of misfolded proteins, as occurs in Creutzfeldt–Jakob disease. Recent work by Desplats and colleagues has suggested that neuronal cells overexpressing α-synuclein could change their conformation and spread from cell to cell. They suggest that in future, treatment directed at specific misfolding of α-synuclein may offer a possible therapeutic strategy for Parkinson's disease.

Presymptomatic duration. There are several hypotheses concerning the length of the presymptomatic (prodromal) phase of Parkinson's disease, which is marked by olfactory loss, autonomic dysfunction (in particular constipation), affective disorders and rapid eye movement sleep behavior disorder (RBD).

- There may be a very long presymptomatic period, spanning two or three decades (Hawkes suggests a presymptomatic period of at least 20 years); it is even possible that a static insult at some point in a person's life may predispose them to develop Parkinson's disease because of the attrition of dopamine-bearing neurons with age.

- Microglial proliferation: there is some evidence from PET scans of microglial activation in people with RBD who are thought to be in the presymptomatic stages of Parkinson's disease. Additionally, microglial proliferation has been found postmortem in people with Parkinson's disease, suggesting ongoing neuronal death. This may mean the presymptomatic period is short.

- Imaging studies using longitudinal fluorodopa-uptake measurements demonstrate a short presymptomatic period. Fluorodopa uptake declines at a rate of about 10% per year in Parkinson's disease; the decline is most rapid in the early stages of the disease. The change is also more rapid in akinetic-rigid patients

25

than in those with tremor-dominant disease, and in patients with young-onset as opposed to old-age-onset Parkinson's disease. Accordingly, it is possible that the presymptomatic period is as short as 5–6 years.

Presymptomatic detection. Individuals with a family history of Parkinson's disease, and those with RBD and impaired olfaction (late-onset hyposmia), may have a higher risk of developing the disease. Major depression, apathy, fatigue, visual impairment, RBD events, erectile dysfunction and pain have also been identified as possible prodromal markers. In the future, it may be possible to recognize individuals who are at risk and initiate neuropreventive therapy. Excessive daytime sleepiness and constipation have also been identified as risk factors. In a 2-year study, 10% of these high-risk individuals showed deterioration in dopaminergic markers, and some developed clinical disease. A large study (the Parkinson's Associated Risk Study [PARS]), involving 7500 relatives of patients with Parkinson's disease, is under way to confirm these findings.

Pathophysiology

Nigral degeneration results in loss of dopamine in the nigrostriatal tract. Nigrostriatal dopaminergic transmission influences motor function through a complex route involving parallel circuits, some of which are inhibitory while others are facilitatory (Figure 2.6). The final common pathway of movement is the motor unit that is influenced through many cortical, reticulospinal and corticospinal tracts. The striatum influences the supplementary motor area through its connections with the ventrolateral nucleus of the thalamus.

The striatal output uses γ-aminobutyric acid (GABA) and is entirely inhibitory. The striatum projects to the medial globus pallidus via two pathways, one indirect and the other direct. Dopamine is inhibitory to the indirect striatopallidal pathway, which first projects to the lateral globus pallidus. The lateral globus pallidus in turn sends another inhibitory projection to the subthalamic nucleus, using GABA as a neurotransmitter. The subthalamic nucleus sends an excitatory glutamatergic output to the medial globus pallidus. Dopamine is excitatory via the D_1 receptors to the direct striatopallidal pathway.

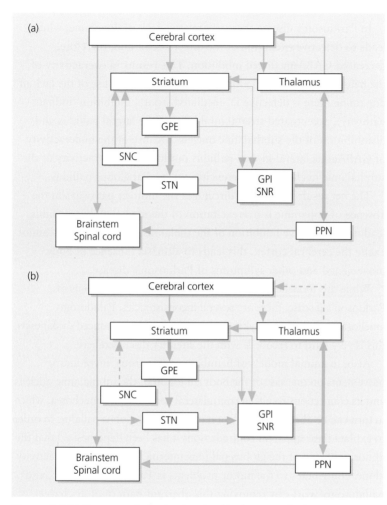

Figure 2.6 (a) The normal circuitry involved in the control of movement, in which the direct pathway (via the globus pallidus interna [(GPI]) and the indirect pathway (via the globus pallidus externa [GPE] and subthalamic nucleus [STN]) are in balance, producing optimal excitation of the thalamus and, thereafter, the cerebral cortex. (b) In Parkinson's disease, there is progressive loss of dopaminergic input from the substantia nigra (SNC) to the striatum, resulting in an imbalance between the direct and indirect pathways, with overactivity of the indirect pathway; overinhibition of the thalamus results in slow and reduced movement. PPN, pedunculopontine nucleus; SNR, substantia nigra reticulata.

27

In Parkinson's disease there is a relative lack of dopamine, which leads to defective excitation of the direct circuit and, therefore, decreased GABA-mediated inhibition. This results in overactivity of the neurons of the medial globus pallidus. Also, because of the lack of dopamine there is defective D_2-mediated striatal inhibition (indirect pathway), accentuated striatal inhibition of the lateral pallidus and disinhibition of the subthalamic nucleus because of the underactivity of GABAergic lateral-globus-pallidus outflow. The overactivity of the subthalamic nucleus then overexcites the medial globus pallidus.

The net result of both the direct and the indirect pathways in the absence of dopamine is overexcitation of the medial globus pallidus, leading to excessive inhibition of the thalamus. If the thalamus cannot excite the cerebral cortex, this leads to akinesia (absence of body movements) and other symptoms of Parkinson's disease.

While this model explains many of the signs and symptoms of Parkinson's disease, there are several inconsistencies. Pallidotomy ameliorates not only bradykinesia but also levodopa-induced dyskinesias; this is very hard to reconcile with the circuitry discussed here.

Also, in animal models of hemiballism (vigorous, involuntary movements on one side of the body), a lesion of the subthalamic nucleus and its connections results in contralateral hemiballism/hemichorea, which in turn can be abolished by a lesion of the medial globus pallidus. In order to explain these apparent contradictions it has been hypothesized that the abnormal firing of the globus pallidus interna, rather than overactivity alone, contributes to the motor problems in Parkinson's disease, and pallidotomy works by removing this aberrant pattern of discharge.

Latest thinking. It is now widely believed that the clinical symptoms of Parkinson's disease are not only due to the loss of a single monoamine neurotransmitter, dopamine, but also the effects of widespread Lewy body disease. This results in a convergence of deficits in multiple transmitter pathways, including the cholinergic, noradrenergic and serotonergic systems, which underpin many of the non-motor symptoms that are integral to Parkinson's disease (Figure 2.7). In addition, glial pathology, neuroimmune responses and proinflammatory cytokines are likely to play a key pathogenic role.

Non-motor symptoms that become evident in the prodromal phase of the disease, such as late-onset hyposmia, RBD, constipation and depression, are all risk factors for Parkinson's disease. Forebrain cholinergic system dysfunction is present in non-demented Parkinson's disease and worsens with dementia.

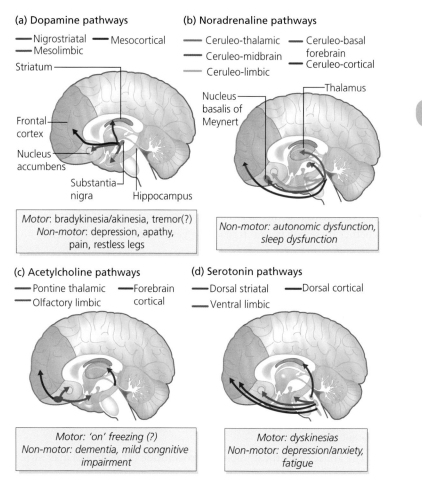

Figure 2.7 Parkinson's disease is a multisystem/multineurotransmitter dysfunction-related disorder. The involvement of multiple neurotransmitters gives rise to the non-motor symptoms of Parkinson's disease, which are driven by both dopaminergic and non-dopaminergic mechanisms.

29

Risk factors

Although Parkinson's disease was first described nearly 200 years ago, it is still impossible to define exactly which individuals are at risk. The aging process is intricately related to the development of Parkinson's disease but is not solely responsible, as some patients develop the disease early in life. Furthermore, the type of dopamine-cell loss in normal aging differs from that in Parkinson's disease. Certain personality traits and environmental factors may increase the risk of Parkinson's disease developing. People with a family history of Parkinson's disease are also at higher risk of developing the disease (see Genetics, pages 31–5).

Personality traits. Patients with certain personality traits, in particular those who are very disciplined and have a tendency to be shy and occasionally depressive, may have a higher risk of developing Parkinson's disease. Such patients usually do not abuse alcohol or cigarettes; it is possible that the apparent protective effects of smoking may be due to nicotine or other tobacco compounds. It is not clear whether these behavioral traits are a genuine risk factor or merely an early indication of dopamine deficiency.

Environmental factors implicated in the genesis of Parkinson's disease include toxins such as herbicides and pesticides (e.g. rotenone). A few studies have found consumption of well water to be a risk factor, and Parkinson's disease seems to be more common in farming communities. Several infectious agents (Table 2.1) or contaminants (heavy metals) have been implicated in the development of syndromes similar to Parkinson's disease; for example, exposure to the manganese found in welding fumes has been suggested as a risk factor (see below).

The abuse of methcathinone hydrochloride (Ephedrone) may also lead to a manganese-induced parkinsonism, possibly accompanied by a mixed hyperkinetic-hypokinetic dysarthria. This has been reported in drug-addicted people from Russia, Ukraine and Estonia, presenting with a levodopa-resistant parkinsonism.

TABLE 2.1

Pathogenic organisms implicated in the causation of (rare) conditions resembling Parkinson's disease

HIV

Nocardia asteroides

Japanese encephalitis virus

Influenza A virus

Helicobacter pylori

Toxoplasma gondii

Prion protein

From Dhawan V, Chaudhuri KR. Parkinson's disease and related disorders part I. In: Koller W, Melamed E, eds. *Handbook of Clinical Neurology.* Amsterdam: Elsevier, 2007:373–84.

A theory for environmental causation was boosted when the use of an illicit drug, MPTP, a by-product of pethidine synthesis, resulted in a mini-epidemic of an illness similar to Parkinson's disease in young people who were abusing the drug intravenously. MPTP destroyed dopamine neurons in the substantia nigra of those affected. The condition responded to dopa drugs in the same way as Parkinson's disease, but Lewy body inclusions were not detected postmortem.

Welding-related parkinsonism. Rare cases of parkinsonism have been linked with exposure to welding fumes, but there is no conclusive evidence that welding either causes parkinsonism or accelerates the onset of Parkinson's disease. Although a community study found higher rates of parkinsonism among welders, controlled epidemiological studies have failed to show that welding is a risk factor for the development of Parkinson's disease.

Genetics

To date, the mechanisms by which genetic changes alter the risk of Parkinson's disease are not fully understood. Research in living human cells is crucial to identify these associations and find new effective targets for disease-modifying treatments.

Genetic investigation of Parkinson's disease is complicated by the same factors that influence the study of its epidemiology. Up to 25% of cases diagnosed as idiopathic Parkinson's disease may actually be some other form of atypical parkinsonism. The familial patterns of Parkinson's disease can be masked if affected family members die before clinical signs become apparent. As Parkinson's disease usually manifests late in life, there are very few affected families with living members from more than two generations. Despite these limitations, significant progress has been made in our understanding of the genetics of the disease from familial aggregation studies, examination of large kindreds and studies in twins.

Familial risk. Individuals with a positive family history have twice the risk of developing Parkinson's disease symptoms. The risk for siblings is increased significantly if there is an affected sibling with young-onset Parkinson's disease. The risk increases further to 12–24% if both a sibling and a parent are affected.

The glucocerebrosidase gene confers susceptibility to the classic Parkinson's disease phenotype in the heterozygous state. Homozygous cases have Gaucher's disease, and typically appear in the Ashkenazi Jewish population.

Large kindred studies. Several families with Parkinson's disease or atypical parkinsonism have been described. A landmark study, initially reported by Golbe et al., of a family who had migrated to New Jersey, USA, from Contursi, Italy, suggested an autosomal-dominant inheritance pattern with high penetrance (i.e. a high frequency of Parkinson's disease among family members with the same genotype). There has been pathological confirmation of Lewy bodies in some family members. Genetic linkage studies have shown that the abnormal gene α-synuclein (*SNCA*) is located on chromosome 4 (Table 2.2) and encodes the protein α-synuclein. Subsequently, the mutation was found to be a substitution of threonine for alanine. How the mutation leads to nigral degeneration and Lewy body formation is unclear. Lewy bodies stain positively for α-synuclein, and α-synuclein aggregation leads to fibril formation. Wszolek et al. identified another large family

TABLE 2.2

Genes/loci implicated in inherited parkinsonism

Symbol	Inheritance	Gene	Location
PARK1	AD	*SNCA* (synuclein alpha)	4q21
PARK2	AR	*Parkin* (parkin RBR E3 ubiquitin protein ligase)	6q25.2–q27
PARK3	AD	Unknown	2p13
PARK5	AD	*UCHL1* (ubiquitin carboxyterminal hydrolase L1)	4p13
PARK6	AR	*PINK1* (phosphatase and tensin homolog-induced putative kinase 1)	1p36
PARK7	AR	DJ-1 protein	1p36
PARK8	AD	*LRRK2* (leucine-rich repeat kinase 2)	12q12
PARK9	AR	ATPase type 13A2 (also known as Kufor–Rakeb syndrome)	1p36
PARK10	Risk factor	Unknown	1p32
PARK11	AD	*GIGYF2* (GRB10 interacting GYF protein 2)	2q37.1
PARK12	Risk factor	Unknown	Xq21–q25
PARK13	AD Risk factor	*HTRA2* (HtrA serine peptidase 2)	2p12
PARK14	AR	*PLA2G6* (phospholipase A2, group 6)	22q13.1
PARK15	AR	*FBXO7* (F-box only protein 7)	22q12–q13
PARK16	Risk factor	Unknown	1q32
PARK17	AD	*VPS35* (VPS35 retromer complex component)	16q11.2
PARK18	AD	*EIF4G1* (eukaryotic translation initiation factor 4 gamma 1)	3q27.1
?	AR	Glucocerebrosidase	1q21

For more information on the genes listed, go to www.ncbi.nlm.nih.gov/gene
AD, autosomal dominant; AR, autosomal recessive; Parkin, Parkinson protein 2.

with 18 affected members within four generations. The gene identified in this kindred, *PARK3*, has been mapped to chromosome 2p13.

However, the *SNCA* and *PARK3* mutations have not been found in many families with autosomal-dominant Parkinson's disease or sporadic Parkinson's disease. Other mutations are being discovered elsewhere (see Table 2.2); mutation in *PARK7* is linked to autosomal-recessive early-onset Parkinson's disease, and was identified in a Dutch and an Italian family, while leucine-rich repeat kinase (*LRRK2*; also known as *PARK8*), with a locus on chromosome 12, was identified in a Japanese family (see below).

Autosomal-recessive juvenile parkinsonism has been studied mainly in Japan. The gene associated with juvenile parkinsonism, *PARK2*, has been mapped to chromosome 6q. The same genetic mutation has been found in European families in individuals with juvenile or young-onset Parkinson's disease. *PARK2* has a 30% homology with the gene that encodes ubiquitin, and is expressed in various regions of the brain (including the substantia nigra) and in liver, heart, testis and skeletal muscle. *PARK2* encodes parkinson protein 2, E3 ubiquitin protein ligase (parkin), which is involved in protein degradation. The *PARK2* mutation appears to lead to defective protein ubiquination, leading to protein aggregation and cell death.

Recent findings in the genetics of Parkinson's disease include the identification of mutations in *LRRK2*, which is involved in mitochondrial functioning, the powerhouse of cells.

LRRK2 is part of the Roco family of genes. Mutation in *LRRK2* has been associated with familial late-onset Parkinson's disease and a few cases of sporadic late-onset Parkinson's disease. The phenotype appears to be identical to sporadic Parkinson's disease, but is associated with behavioral disorders, leg tremor, sleep disturbances and slight cognitive decline. One case of an Ile1371Val substitution in *LRRK2* has been reported, with the typical Lewy body pathology that stained positive for ubiquitin and α-synuclein and symptoms identical to idiopathic sporadic Parkinson's disease. The most common *LRRK2* substitution is Gly2019Ser, which accounts for 2% of sporadic and 5% of familial cases. This substitution is identified more frequently in

North African Arabs and Ashkenazi Jews, while a Gly2385Arg mutation has been described in the Chinese/Taiwanese population.

Previously identified genes have been pivotal to understanding the process of neurodegeneration. However, the clinical impact of these gene mutations has been limited because they are usually identified in patients with early-onset Parkinson's disease (e.g. with *PARK2* and *PINK1* [also known as *PARK6*]) or with atypical parkinsonism (as with *MAPT*).

In the genome-wide scan for Parkinson's disease (GenePD) study, which investigated the effect of heterozygous *PARK2* mutations on age of onset in patients with familial Parkinson's disease, one member from each of 183 families was screened for *PARK2* mutations: 12.6% of the families were positive. Of these, 43% were compound heterozygotes, 13% were homozygotes and 10% were heterozygotes. The age of onset of Parkinson's disease was significantly lower in those with one *PARK2* mutation than in those with none (11.7 years earlier), and also significantly lower in those with two mutations than in those with one (13.2 years earlier). The study showed that the *PARK2* mutation is not rare, and that heterozygosity significantly lowers the age of onset of Parkinson's disease. Clinically, however, it is not possible to distinguish between patients with a *Parkin-*, *PINK1-* and *DJ-1*-linked form of Parkinson's disease.

Studies in twins have been performed since 1967. Ward et al. studied 43 monozygotic and 19 dizygotic pairs of twins, and found that the concordance rate for parkinsonism was no more frequent in twins than expected, given the general rate of disease. They concluded that the main causative factors are probably not genetic. However, Parkinson's disease may be asymptomatic in the unaffected twin. Burn et al. studied 18-fluorodopa PET scans in sets of twins in which one of each pair had clinical Parkinson's disease. The clinically unaffected twin frequently had abnormally low 18-fluorodopa uptake. Follow-up of some of the twins revealed worsening of this abnormality, suggesting progressive deterioration of nigrostriatal function. The PET findings suggested concordance rates of 45% for monozygotic and 29% for dizygotic twins. Therefore, it seems that some genetic contribution to Parkinson's disease is likely.

Key points – epidemiology, pathophysiology and genetics

- Parkinson's disease is one of the most common neurodegenerative diseases, with a prevalence of approximately 200 per 100 000 individuals.
- The incidence and prevalence of Parkinson's disease increases sharply with age.
- Men are 1.5 times more likely than women to develop the disease.
- Pathologically, Parkinson's disease is characterized by widespread neurodegeneration including that of neuromelanin-containing neurons, as well as deficits in the serotonergic, cholinergic and noradrenergic systems that result in the manifestation of motor and non-motor symptoms. Lewy bodies in the remaining nigral neurons are a pathological hallmark of the disease after death.
- The cause of neuronal degeneration is uncertain.
- Braak has suggested that the condition may begin in the olfactory bundle and lower brainstem, and studies are under way to identify specific non-motor biomarkers of the prodromal phase of Parkinson's disease.
- Rapid eye movement behavior disorder (RBD), late-onset hyposmia, constipation and major depression are all risk factors for Parkinson's disease.
- At present, there are no guidelines for genetic testing in Parkinson's disease. Genetic tests for common mutations such as *LRRK2* Gly2019Ser mutations in at-risk individuals (European, North African and Ashkenazi Jewish), glucocerebrosidase (*GBA*) mutations, or *Parkin* (autosomal recessive) are usually available if they are thought to be clinically relevant and necessary. Where possible, advice from a genetic counselor must be obtained before genetic testing.

Key references

Berger K, Breteler MM, Helmer C et al. Prognosis with Parkinson's disease in Europe: a collaborative study of population-based cohorts. Neurologic Diseases in the Elderly Research Group. *Neurology* 2000;54(suppl 5):S24–7.

Braak H, Del Tredici K, Rüb U et al. Staging of brain pathology related to sporadic Parkinson's disease. *Neurobiol Aging* 2003;24:197–211.

Braak H, Ghebremedhin E, Rub U et al. Stages in the development of Parkinson's disease-related pathology. *Cell Tissue Res* 2004; 318:121–34.

Burn DJ, Mark MH, Playford ED et al. Parkinson's disease in twins studied with 18F-dopa and positron emission tomography. *Neurology* 1992;42:1894–900.

Desplats P, Lee HJ, Bae EJ et al. Inclusion formation and neuronal cell death through neuron-to-neuron transmission of alpha-synuclein. *Proc Natl Acad Sci USA* 2009; 106:13010–15.

Diamond SG, Markham CH, Hoehn MM et al. Effect of age at onset on progression and mortality in Parkinson's disease. *Neurology* 1989;39:1187–90.

Foltynie T, Sawcer S, Brayne C, Barker RA. The genetic basis of Parkinson's disease. *J Neurol Neurosurg Psychiatry* 2002;73: 363–70.

Gao X, Chen H, Schwarzschild MA et al. Erectile function and risk of Parkinson's disease. *Am J Epidemiol* 2007;166:1446–50.

Giordana MT, D'Agostino C, Albani G et al. Neuropathology of Parkinson's disease associated with the *LRRK2* Ile1371Val mutation. *Mov Disord* 2007;22:275–8.

Golbe LI, Di Iorio G, Sanges G et al. Clinical genetic analysis of Parkinson's disease in the Contursi kindred. *Ann Neurol* 1996;40: 767–75.

Hawkes CH, Del Tredici K, Braak H. Parkinson's disease: a dual hit hypothesis. *Neuropath Appl Neurobiol* 2007;33:599–614.

Hely MA, Morris JG, Reid WG et al. Age at onset: the major determinant of outcome in Parkinson's disease. *Acta Neurol Scand* 1995;92:455–63.

Hoehn MM, Yahr MD. Parkinsonism: onset, progression, and mortality. *Neurology* 1998;50:318 (reprinted from *Neurology* 1967;17:427–42).

Jennings D, Siderowf A, Stern M et al. Evaluating phenoconversion to PD in the PARS prodromal cohort. *Mov Disord* 2013;28(suppl1): abstr. 152.

Khan NL, Jain S, Lynch JM et al. Mutations in the gene *LRRK2* encoding dardarin (*PARK8*) cause familial Parkinson's disease: clinical, pathological, olfactory and functional imaging and genetic data. *Brain* 2005;128:2786–96.

Klein C, Westenberger A. Genetics of Parkinson's disease. *Cold Spring Harb Perspect Med* 2012;2:a008888.

Lin CH, Wu RM, Chang HY et al. Preceding pain symptoms and Parkinson's disease: a nationwide population-based cohort study. *Eur J Neurol* 2013;20:1398–404.

Mata IF, Ross OA, Kachergus J et al. *LRRK2* mutations are a common cause of Parkinson's disease in Spain. *Eur J Neurol* 2006;13:391–4.

Olanow CW, Prusiner SB. Is Parkinson's disease a prion disorder? *Proc Natl Acad Sci USA* 2009;106: 12571–2.

Sheerin U-M, Houlden H, Wood NW. Advances in the genetics of Parkinson's disease: a guide for the clinician. *Mov Disord Clin Pract* 2014;1:3–13.

Sixel-Döring F, Trautmann E, Mollenhauer B, Trenkwalder C. Rapid eye movement sleep behavioral events: a new marker for neurodegeneration in early Parkinson's Disease? *Sleep* 2014;37:431–8.

Sun M, Latourelle JC, Wooten GF et al. Influence of heterozygosity for *Parkin* mutation on onset age in familial Parkinson disease: the GenePD study. *Arch Neurol* 2006; 63:826–32.

Tanner CM, Brandabur M, Dorsey ER. Parkinson disease: a global view. *Parkinson Report* Spring 2008, 9–11.

Ward CD, Duvoisin RC, Ince SE et al. Parkinson's disease in 65 pairs of twins and in a set of quadruplets. *Neurology* 1983;33:815–24.

Wszolek ZK, Pfeiffer B, Fulgham JR et al. Western Nebraska family (family D) with autosomal dominant parkinsonism. *Neurology* 1995;45: 502–5.

When, in 1817, James Parkinson first described the features of
paralysis agitans in 6 patients, he did not refer to the typical cogwheel
rigidity, and mistook bradykinesia for paralysis. Nevertheless, his
description of the tremor, posture (Figure 3.1) and clinical course of
the disease has stood the test of time and remains valid today. Most
cases of Parkinson's disease are easily recognizable at an early stage,
but many are missed if tremor is absent; gradual slowing in
performance may be instead attributed to aging or aches and pains,
and loss of function may be ascribed to other causes.

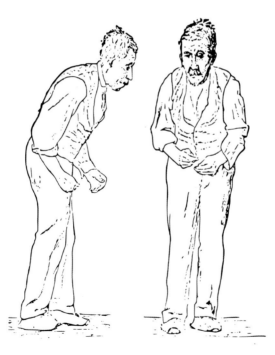

Figure 3.1 Paralysis agitans, as first described by James Parkinson,
depicting the characteristic fixed posture. Neurologist Sir William Richard
Gowers drew this illustration in 1886 as part of his documentation of
Parkinson's disease in *A Manual of Diseases of the Nervous System*.

Parkinsonism is a clinical syndrome (Table 3.1) and may have a number of causes. When the condition appears to be idiopathic and, in particular, responds to levodopa therapy, it is referred to as Parkinson's disease.

Early motor and non-motor indicators

Signs may be subtle in the early stages of the disease. In suspected cases it is often helpful to ask patients what tasks they find difficult.

TABLE 3.1

Features that support a diagnosis of parkinsonism

Essential features

- Bradykinesia and one (or more) of the following:
  - tremor (resting)
  - rigidity (cogwheel or lead-pipe; see page 46)
  - postural instability

Additional motor features

- Fixed, stooped posture
- Dystonic postures, e.g. striatal hand, striatal toe
- Hypomimia ('masked' face)
- Shuffling, short-step gait (with or without festination)
- Freezing episodes (sometimes known as paradoxical akinesia)

Additional non-motor features

- Late-onset hyposmia
- Depression and anxiety
- Constipation
- Bladder symptoms
- Pain (usually unilateral on the affected side)
- Subtle mental and cognitive disturbance (mild cognitive impairment)

"So what drove me to the doctor? Initially it was a stiff shoulder, but mainly it was my handwriting. In 6 months it had changed from elegant script to scrawl"

Motor indicators

- Dressing or other activities requiring fine finger movements may become awkward and take longer than usual.
- Swinging of arms, an automatic movement, may become impaired on the side affected by Parkinson's disease.
- Walking in crowds may be difficult, because the person cannot make the rapid adjustments necessary to avoid bumping into other people.
- Getting out of a low chair can be problematic (although the patient may have noticed this, they may be unable to explain why it is difficult).
- Handwriting often deteriorates, with the writing typically becoming smaller; if the patient is asked to draw a spiral this will be smaller than that drawn by the doctor or nurse in the clinic (Figure 3.2). Comparison of the patient's writing from the past with that drawn in the clinic may be useful.
- Facial expression becomes impassive and the patient may blink infrequently; this mask-like expression can conceal the patient's normal thoughts and emotions.

(a) (b) (c)

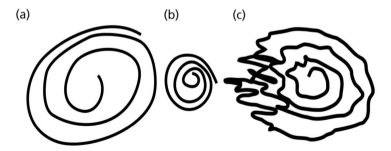

Figure 3.2 Spiral drawings may help to differentiate between parkinsonian and essential tremor. When asked to replicate a spiral (a) drawn by the doctor or nurse, a patient with (b) parkinsonian tremor is likely to produce a much smaller version, whereas a patient with (c) essential tremor will produce a shakier but similar-sized version of the original.

- Speech may be soft and low in volume, with frequent pauses. Patients may have difficulty enunciating syllables and words separately, so the sounds become merged and speech may be difficult to understand.

Non-motor indicators

- There may be a very early loss or impaired sense of smell. In the absence of any other causes of loss of smell, late-onset hyposmia may herald the development of Parkinson's disease.
- Specific sleep disorders such as rapid eye movement (REM) behavior disorder (RBD) may develop.
- Major depression, cognitive dysfunction, falls and/or constipation may accompany RBD or hyposmia.
- Specific color blindness and contrast sensitivity may develop.

Symptoms and signs

There are several prodromal imaging possibilities such as diffusion-weighted (MR) imaging (DWI) of the olfactory tract, [^{123}I] meta-iodobenzylguanidine (MIBG) single-photon emission computed tomography (SPECT), dopamine transporter SPECT, [^{18}F]-dopa positron emission tomography (PET) and transcranial sonography.

Tremor is an approximately rhythmic and roughly sinusoidal involuntary movement of part(s) of the body as a result of repetitive muscle contractions. The presence of an obvious tremor often leads both patients and their carers to suspect Parkinson's disease. Parkinsonian tremor is worse at rest (4–7 Hz) and is often unilateral. It affects 70% of patients with Parkinson's disease and is the presenting feature in most cases. However, those presenting with akinetic-rigid parkinsonism may never have significant tremor.

> *"Certainly in the initial stages of disease this was the most embarrassing of my symptoms. The tremor was mainly in my left arm and became worse as I became more embarrassed or stressed. I used to deal with it by sitting on my left hand."*

Tremor often has a rotary component that is almost always indicative of Parkinson's disease; for example, patients may be seen 'pill rolling', the action of rolling a small sphere between thumb and index finger. Some have emergent tremor, i.e. tremor that appears after an initial delay.

Parkinsonian versus essential tremor. Parkinsonian tremor does not interfere with activity, whereas essential tremor is postural and affects function, such as carrying a cup of tea, often causing the patient to spill drinks. In addition, alcohol may attenuate essential tremor in some cases, but this type of response is unusual with parkinsonian tremor.

It is important to differentiate essential tremor from parkinsonian tremor (see Figure 3.2), as the former carries a more benign prognosis and is twice as common, with a prevalence of at least 400 per 100 000 (Table 3.2). Parkinsonian tremor, while worrying and embarrassing for the patient, is generally a good sign in Parkinson's disease because it can presage a more benign course. However, the tremor itself may only partially respond to dopaminergic therapy.

Dystonic tremor. Some patients diagnosed with essential tremor may actually have dystonic tremor, which is associated with dystonic posturing of the limb. The natural history of this condition remains unclear. Such patients may be misdiagnosed with Parkinson's disease, but DaTSCAN (see page 56) is usually normal in these cases.

Bradykinesia/akinesia is difficulty in initiating, and slowness in executing, movement. It is the most disabling motor manifestation of Parkinson's disease. It first affects fine movements such as fastening buttons and handwriting, which starts normal sized but becomes smaller and more cramped and may progressively tail off (micrographia). One or both arms may stop swinging when walking.

Later, gait is affected, with difficulty starting off walking, small steps and shuffling. 'Festination' describes the typical hurrying gait, which may be interrupted by sudden stops as if the patient is nailed to the floor. Carers may nudge patients to start them moving again. These freezing episodes (paroxysmal akinesia) are often provoked by visual stimuli, such as an open doorway, or by anxiety. Many patients develop tricks to overcome the symptom, such as stepping over an inverted walking stick or marching to a rhythm. Eventually, some but

43

TABLE 3.2

Comparison of parkinsonian, essential and dystonic tremor

Feature	Parkinsonian tremor	Essential tremor	Dystonic tremor
Age at onset	Usually > 50 years	Any age	Young adulthood (20–30 years) or older (50–70 years)
Family history	Unusual	Common	'Dystonia gene-associated tremor'
Site	Usually hands, also legs and jaw; head (uncommon)	Hands, head (a no–no or yes–yes motion), vocal cords, tongue; legs (rare)	Usually limbs or head (torticollis), hands (writer's cramp), and vocal cords (uncommon)
Characteristics	At rest; reduced by supination/pronation action; increased by mental concentration	Postural; increased by flexion/extension action	Appears with dystonia; may temporarily disappear with a sensory trick, at rest, in sustained postures and in voluntary movement
Frequency (Hz)	4–7	8–12	Irregular (mainly < 7)
Lead-pipe rigidity*	Yes	No	No
Cogwheel rigidity*	Yes	Rare	No
Alcohol	No effect	Often improves	Often improves, can lead to rebound
Treatment	Dopaminergics[†] Anticholinergics[‡]	β-blockers, primidone (use with caution)	Botulinum toxin injection, trihexyphenidyl, benzodiazepines

*See page 46. [†]Levodopa may be more effective than dopamine agonists.
[‡]No longer recommended.

> *"I have only started to experience these symptoms in the last few months and find them more embarrassing than the tremor. Trying to fasten/unfasten buttons on a shirt or a trouser fly, or to tie shoe laces, can be very frustrating, particularly when at other times of the day I'm 'back to normal' and do not have any problems."*

not all patients require a wheelchair; however, in the early stages of disease, this is a red flag for an atypical parkinsonian syndrome and the diagnosis should be reappraised.

Other signs of bradykinesia include characteristic facial impassivity (hypomimia), which, if unilateral, may be misinterpreted as facial paralysis. Speech may assume a quiet monotonous character. A clinical clue is fatiguing or 'pauses' while performing a repetitive movement such as finger tapping or clenching and unclenching of the fist.

Sensors worn on the wrist, ankle or trunk, are now available to objectively measure off periods, bradykinesia and dyskinesia (Figure 3.3). These will improve objective measurement of motor symptoms. Recent studies also indicate that the Parkinson's Kinetigraph (PKG) may provide valuable information on sleep function, particularly if patients suddenly doze off, increasing the risk of driving accidents.

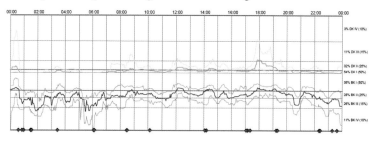

Figure 3.3 Standard Parkinson's Kinetigraph (PKG) report. The green tracing indicates dyskinesia, the blue tracing indicates bradykinesia and the red diamonds show the times at which medication was taken. Reports such as this provide clinicians with an objective measure of the motor syndrome such that they can alter the amount or frequency of medication or recommend a new therapy as appropriate.

Rigidity is defined as increased resistance to passive movement; it is therefore a clinical sign detected by physicians. However, patients often complain of muscular stiffness and pain, which may be diffuse or localized to one limb or the trunk. Parkinsonian rigidity is detected by moving the body part slowly and gently (in contrast to the quick movement needed to elicit spasticity of pyramidal origin). Parkinsonian rigidity, which can be activated by asking the patient to perform movements in the opposite limb (Froment sign, synkinesis or reinforcement), presents as one of two types:
- 'lead-pipe' rigidity – a constant resistance to passive movement
- 'cogwheel' rigidity – a superimposed clicking resistance (like a ratchet), which has been attributed to underlying tremor.

Postural problems. The bent posture of Parkinson's disease is probably due to rigidity and muscle spasm, although other factors may contribute. In some, this may become dominant (camptocormia). In others, there may be a tendency for the trunk to sway to one side ('Pisa' syndrome) (Figure 3.4).

Flexion is encountered particularly in the neck and trunk, and also when the arms are brought forward in front of the body. Additional flexion at the hips and knees may lead to walking on tiptoe (simian gait) in fully developed disease.

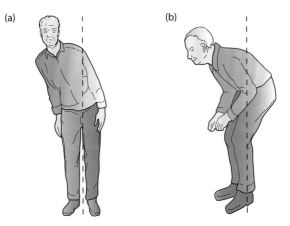

Figure 3.4 (a) Pisa syndrome is characterized by lateral flexion of the trunk. (b) Camptocormia is characterized by forward flexion of the spine.

Postural imbalance can be detected by the 'pull' test. The doctor stands behind the patient and applies a quick pull backwards to the front of the shoulders. Parkinsonian patients typically fall backwards or totter without corrective action, leading to a fall 'en bloc' (in one piece).

Falls are common in late Parkinson's disease and are a major cause of morbidity. They may be due to postural imbalance, a displaced center of gravity, freezing of gait and/or failure to detect displacement and take corrective action.

Non-motor-symptoms. A wide range of non-motor symptoms has been described in Parkinson's disease, all of which are likely to have a major effect on the health-related quality of life of patients. These symptoms include depression, dementia, sleep disorders, bowel and bladder problems, fatigue, apathy, pain and autonomic dysfunction (Table 3.3). Non-motor symptoms are common and can occur at all stages of the disease, even before diagnosis (prodromal phase) (Table 3.4).

Before any drug treatment is started, more than 45% of patients may show a severe to very severe burden of non-motor symptoms regardless of motor impairment. Despite this, non-motor symptoms tend to be poorly recognized by health professionals, who tend to focus on motor symptoms.

The development and validation of instruments such as the Non-Motor Symptom (NMS) Questionnaire (NMSQuest; Figure 3.5), the NMS Scale (NMSS), the SCOPA (SCale for Outcome in PArkinson's disease), and the Movement Disorder Society's Unified Parkinson's Disease Rating Scale (MDS-UPDRS) has helped to make comprehensive evaluation of non-motor symptoms possible in patients with Parkinson's disease. National and international societies such as the UK Department of Health, the International Movement Disorders Society and the US National Institute of Neurological Disorders and Stroke, as well as patient groups such as Parkinson's UK recommend giving patients the NMSQuest to fill out as a matter of routine while they are waiting to be seen by a clinician.

Figure 3.6 outlines a plan for routine use of the NMSQuest in clinical practice.

TABLE 3.3

The range of non-motor symptoms in Parkinson's disease* using validated tools such as the NMSQuest (see Figure 3.5)

Neuropsychiatric symptoms

- Major depression
- Anxiety
- Hallucinations, delusions, illusions
- Delirium (may be drug induced)
- Cognitive impairment (dementia, MCI)
- Dopamine dysregulation syndrome (usually related to levodopa)
- Impulse control disorders (related to dopaminergic drugs)
- Panic attacks (could be 'off' related)

Sleep disorders and dysfunctions

- REM sleep behavior disorder (possibly prodromal)
- Excessive daytime sleepiness, narcolepsy-type 'sleep attack'
- Restless legs syndrome, periodic leg movements
- Insomnia (onset and maintenance)
- Sleep disordered breathing
- Non-REM parasomnias (confusional wandering, sleep talking)

Fatigue

- Central fatigue (may be related to dysautonomia)
- Peripheral fatigue

Sensory symptoms

- Parkinsonian pain (Chaudhuri–Schapira classification)
  - Musculoskeletal pain
  - PD-related chronic pain (may respond to dopaminergic therapy)
    - ➤ central pain
    - ➤ visceral pain
  - Fluctuation-related pain (responsive to dopaminergic therapy)
    - ➤ dyskinetic pain
    - ➤ 'off' period dystonia-related pain
    - ➤ 'off' period generalized pain
  - Nocturnal pain (usually responsive to dopaminergic therapy)
    - ➤ RLS/PLM-related pain
    - ➤ nocturnal akinesia-linked pain
  - Coat-hanger pain (rare, and linked to postural hypotension)

CONTINUED

TABLE 3.3 (CONTINUED)

- Orofacial pain
  - ➢ temporomandibular joint pain
  - ➢ bruxism-related pain
  - ➢ burning mouth syndrome (may be responsive to levodopa)
- Peripheral limb/abdominal pain
  - ➢ drug-induced
  - ➢ linked to peripheral edema
  - ➢ lower bowel pain related to retroperitoneal fibrosis
- Olfactory disturbance (hyposmia, functional anosmia)

Autonomic dysfunction

- Bladder urgency, frequency, nocturia
- Sexual dysfunction (may be drug-induced)
- Erectile dysfunction
- Sweating abnormalities (hyperhidrosis)
- Orthostatic hypotension, postprandial hypotension

Gastrointestinal symptoms

- Dribbling of saliva
- Dysphagia
- Ageusia (change in sensation to taste)
- Constipation
- *Nausea, vomiting, reflux, fecal incontinence*

Dopaminergic drug-induced – behavioral

- Hallucinations, psychosis, delusions
- Dopamine dysregulation syndrome (usually linked to levodopa intake)
- *Impulse-control disorders (e.g. compulsive gambling, hypersexuality, binge eating)*

Dopaminergic drug-induced – 'other'

- Ankle swelling
- Dyspnea (may be linked to ergot dopamine agonist-related cardiac/respiratory failure)
- Skin reactions
  - subcutaneous nodules (apomorphine)
  - erythematous rash (rotigotine patch)

Symptoms reported during episodes of non-motor fluctuations

- Anxiety/panic attacks
- Drenching sweats
- Dystonic / Nocturnal pain
- Slowness of thinking
- Fatigue
- Akathisia
- Irritability/mood changes
- Hallucinations

CONTINUED

TABLE 3.3 (CONTINUED)

Other symptoms

- *Weight loss (could be an indication of susceptibility to dyskinesia)*
- *Weight gain (could be related to binge eating in impulse-control disorders)*

Visual disturbances

- Retinal origin
- Blue–green color vision impairment (could be a prodromal sign accompanying REM behavior disorder)
- Visual contrast insensitivity
- Dyskinesia/motor fluctuation-related visual contrast super-sensitivity (may lead to blurred vision)

Ocular/sensory problems

- Blepharitis
- Ocular pain
- Ocular fatigue (asthenopenia)
- Xerophthalmos
- Photophobia
- Excessive tearing
- Blurred vision and reading difficulty
- Diplopia (fleeting, fluctuation-related, selective)
- Pupillary problems (impaired response to light and pain)

*On average, a patient with Parkinson's disease expresses 8–12 different non-motor symptoms. Note: symptoms in italics are lesser-known symptoms. MCI, minimal cognitive impairment; PLM, periodic leg movement; REM, rapid eye movement; RLS, restless legs syndrome.

TABLE 3.4

Non-motor symptoms suggestive of Parkinson's disease before diagnosis (prodromal phase)

Strong evidence	Suggested links (poor evidence base)	
• Constipation	• Restless legs syndrome	• Anxiety
• Olfactory deficit (hyposmia)	• Apathy	• Pain
• REM sleep behavior disorder	• Fatigue	• Visual impairment
• Major depression	• Excessive daytime sleepiness	• Erectile dysfunction
		• RBD events

RBD, REM behavior disorder; REM, rapid eye movement.

PD NMS QUESTIONNAIRE

Name: .... Date: .... Age: ....

Centre ID: Male ☐ Female ☐

NON-MOVEMENT PROBLEMS IN PARKINSON'S
The movement symptoms of Parkinson's are well known. However, other problems can sometimes occur as part of the condition or its treatment. It is important that the doctor knows about these, particularly if they are troublesome for you.

A range of problems is listed below. Please tick the box 'Yes' if you have experienced it **during the past month.** The doctor or nurse may ask you some questions to help decide. If you have **not** experienced the problem in the past month tick the 'No' box. You should answer 'No' even if you have had the problem in the past but not in the past month.

Have you experienced any of the following in the last month?

	Yes	No
1. Dribbling of saliva during the daytime	☐	☐
2. Loss or change in your ability to taste or smell	☐	☐
3. Difficulty swallowing food or drink or problems with choking	☐	☐
4. Vomiting or feelings of sickness (nausea)	☐	☐
5. Constipation (less than 3 bowel movements a week) or having to strain to pass a stool (faeces)	☐	☐
6. Bowel (faecal) incontinence	☐	☐
7. Feeling that your bowel emptying is incomplete after having been to the toilet	☐	☐
8. A sense of urgency to pass urine makes you rush to the toilet	☐	☐
9. Getting up regularly at night to pass urine	☐	☐
10. Unexplained pains (not due to known conditions such as arthritis)	☐	☐
11. Unexplained change in weight (not due to change in diet)	☐	☐
12. Problems remembering things that have happened recently or forgetting to do things	☐	☐
13. Loss of interest in what is happening around you or doing things	☐	☐
14. Seeing or hearing things that you know or are told are not there	☐	☐
15. Difficulty concentrating or staying focused	☐	☐

	Yes	No
16. Feeling sad, 'low' or 'blue'	☐	☐
17. Feeling anxious, frightened or panicky	☐	☐
18. Feeling less interested in sex or more interested in sex	☐	☐
19. Finding it difficult to have sex when you try	☐	☐
20. Feeling light headed, dizzy or weak standing from sitting or lying	☐	☐
21. Falling	☐	☐
22. Finding it difficult to stay awake during activities such as working, driving or eating	☐	☐
23. Difficulty getting to sleep at night or staying asleep at night	☐	☐
24. Intense, vivid dreams or frightening dreams	☐	☐
25. Talking or moving about in your sleep as if you are 'acting' out a dream	☐	☐
26. Unpleasant sensations in your legs at night or while resting, and a feeling that you need to move	☐	☐
27. Swelling of your legs	☐	☐
28. Excessive sweating	☐	☐
29. Double vision	☐	☐
30. Believing things are happening to you that other people say are not true	☐	☐

All the information you supply through this form will be treated with confidence and will only be used for the purpose for which it has been collected. Information supplied will be used for monitoring purposes. Your personal data will be processed and held in accordance with the Data Protection Act 1998.

Developed and validated by the International PD Non Motor Group
For information contact: susanne.tluk@uhl.nhs.uk or alison.forbes@uhl.nhs.uk

Figure 3.5 The Non-Motor Symptoms Questionnaire (NMSQuest). Available online at www.pdnmg.com/imagelib/pdf/nms-quest.pdf and at www.parkinsons.org.uk/professionals/resources/non-motor-symptoms-questionnaire. Reproduced with permission from Chaudhuri et al., 2007.

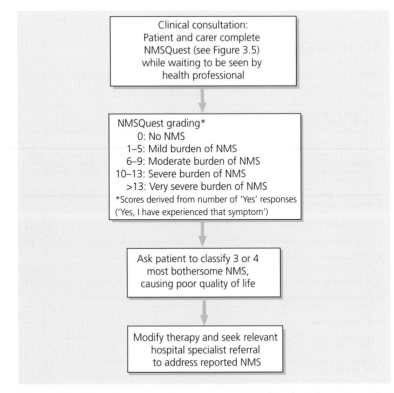

Figure 3.6 Addressing non-motor symptoms (NMS) in clinical practice using the NMSQuest questionnaire (see Figure 3.5).

New diagnostic criteria

The Movement Disorders Society has recently revised the clinical criteria for the diagnosis of Parkinson's disease, incorporating a range of non-motor symptoms as well as retaining the central core motor features. Recognizing that no diagnosis of Parkinson's disease can be made with 100% certainty and that the error rate can range from 75–95%, the new criteria suggest a two-way process: parkinsonism is first defined using central motor symptoms such as bradykinesia, tremor and rigidity; these are then considered with respect to ancillary and non-motor issues to determine whether the motor syndrome is likely to be specific to Parkinson's disease or not.

Criteria for prodromal Parkinson's disease have also been suggested but only for use within a research framework.

Confirmation of diagnosis

The diagnosis of Parkinson's disease remains primarily clinical; there are as yet no specific tests. Dopaminergic challenge tests (see below) are not routinely recommended for diagnostic purposes.

Dopaminergic challenge. The response to levodopa, or to dopaminergic agents such as apomorphine, has been used as a potential diagnostic test for Parkinson's disease but it is fraught with pitfalls. Many Parkinson-plus syndromes such as multiple system atrophy (MSA) and progressive supranuclear palsy (PSP) also respond initially to levodopa or dopaminergic therapy, so **the use of challenge tests for diagnostic purposes is not recommended. There is also concern about the use of levodopa in untreated levodopa-naive patients, since a possible priming action of levodopa for the development of future dyskinesias has been demonstrated in animal models.** The authors stress the importance of the points shown in bold.

Typically, a patient with idiopathic Parkinson's disease will show a significant response to dopaminergic agents; about 50% of patients will go on to develop dyskinesia after 2–5 years of standard therapy with levodopa (at doses exceeding 600 mg/day), although this proportion is lower when smaller doses of levodopa (150–300 mg/day) are given.

Approximately 20% of patients with parkinsonian symptoms exhibit little response to dopaminergic treatment. Many of these have a different underlying disease, such as MSA, PSP, corticobasal degeneration or primary striatonigral degeneration (Table 3.5). Patients who do not respond to levodopa therapy have a worse prognosis, probably with a progressive course and reduced life expectancy.

Imaging tests

CT or MRI scans are usually not needed for diagnosis, but a brain scan should be performed if parkinsonism is purely unilateral or otherwise atypical, or if additional signs (e.g. pyramidal) are present. CT or MRI may also be used to rule out a space-occupying lesion, vascular disease and normal-pressure hydrocephalus. This last condition causes lower-body parkinsonism, cognitive decline and early bladder symptoms.

TABLE 3.5

Reasons to reappraise the diagnosis

- No, incomplete or short-lived response to levodopa
- Early-onset severe bulbar disturbance (speech and swallowing)
- Early-onset balance problems and falls (within 1–2 years of diagnosis)
- Patient is wheelchair bound relatively rapidly (within 5 years of diagnosis)
- Preferential involvement of the lower extremity, with normal upper-extremity function
- Early-onset dementia or hallucinations (within 2 years)
- A prominent eye-movement disorder (supranuclear gaze, palsy, nystagmus)
- Intrusive early-onset autonomic problems
  - bladder symptoms
  - sexual disturbance
  - significant postural hypotension

The use of DWI and diffusion tensor (MR) imaging (DTI) has been explored and developed in an effort to differentiate idiopathic Parkinson's disease from parkinsonism due to other causes such as MSA. DWI reflects a quantifiable coefficient known as the apparent diffusion coefficient (ADC), and preliminary reports suggest that idiopathic Parkinson's disease produces substantially higher regional ADC values than does MSA. DWI is also thought to differentiate between MSA and PSP. Further studies using this potentially widely available technique are under way.

Transcranial ultrasound scanning. In the last decade, there has been considerable interest in using transcranial ultrasound scanning (TCUS) in Parkinson's disease. Using TCUS, several studies, mainly in Austria and Germany, have reported hyperechogenicity (increased size) of the substantia nigra in patients with Parkinson's disease (Figure 3.7). In a study by Berg et al., substantia nigra hyperechogenicity was noted in 103 of 112 patients with clinically diagnosed Parkinson's disease.

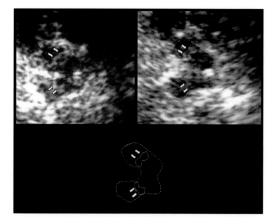

Figure 3.7 Substantia nigra hyperechogenicity on transcranial ultrasound scanning, as outlined here, is a typical marker in Parkinson's disease. Reproduced with permission from Berg D et al. 2005.

To address concerns about the subjective nature of the test and investigator bias, Prestel et al. blinded the sonographer to the clinical diagnosis of 42 patients with Parkinson's disease and 35 controls. This left the diagnosis to be made solely on the basis of substantia nigra hyperechogenicity. The study yielded a positive predictive value of 85.7% and a negative predictive value of 82.9%, suggesting that TCUS may indeed be a useful diagnostic tool for Parkinson's disease.

The substantia nigra hyperechogenicity seen in over 90% of Parkinson's disease patients is thought to reflect increased amounts of iron bound to proteins other than ferritin. No differences in substantia nigra hyperechogenicity have been found in the different clinical subtypes of idiopathic Parkinson's disease. In a longitudinal study by Berg et al., in which patients had an initial examination and then another one 5 years later, the mean (± SD) UPDRS scores changed from 26.3 (± 11.7) to 49.2 (± 21.3). However, there was no corresponding increase in substantia nigra hyperechogenicity, suggesting that this measure does not change with the pathological progression of the disease.

Transcranial ultrasonography is recommended in the EFNS/MDS-ES guidelines to help differentiate between Parkinson's disease and atypical and secondary parkinsonian disorders, as well as for the early diagnosis of Parkinson's disease and for the detection of individuals at risk of developing the disease. However, the technique is still not widely used, possibly because it requires considerable local expertise and training.

Single-photon emission computed tomography (SPECT) with DaTSCAN. DaTSCAN, an ethanolic solution containing a radioiodine-labeled cocaine derivative, is administered intravenously 3–6 hours before imaging by SPECT. The radiopharmaceutical binds with presynaptic dopamine transporters, enabling an assessment of neuronal degeneration to be made (Figure 3.8). SPECT can be used to confirm a positive clinical examination and also to differentiate difficult clinical cases: essential tremor (which is likely to show a normal image) may mimic parkinsonian tremor (which shows an abnormal image). The value of SPECT scanning becomes evident in clinical trials involving patients with suspected Parkinson's disease; 4–14% of them have scans with no dopaminergic deficits. These individuals do not show a progressive decline in dopaminergic markers, suggesting that they do not have Parkinson's disease. This type of imaging also appears to correlate with the progression of Parkinson's disease. However, at present, it is unable to differentiate between Parkinson's disease, MSA and PSP.

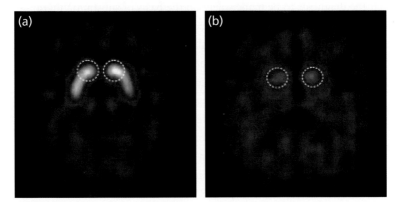

Figure 3.8 SPECT scans using DaTSCAN, showing transverse images of the striatum and uptake of the radiopharmaceutical in dopamine-producing neurons. (a) Characteristic 'comma' shape and circular 'full stop' (as marked) in a normal brain, indicating uptake in the putamen and caudate, respectively. (b) Loss of uptake in the putamen due to Parkinson's disease, although uptake in the caudate (as marked by the circle) is initially preserved. Images courtesy of GE Healthcare.

Other tests. A PET scan with fluorodopa can localize dopamine deficiency in the basal ganglia (see Figure 2.5), while autonomic tests and sphincter electromyography may support a diagnosis of MSA. PET, while more sensitive than SPECT, is only available in research-based studies and is not routinely indicated in clinical practice.

Approximately 10% of individuals thought to have Parkinson's disease may have normal dopaminergic imaging – Subjects Without Evidence of Dopaminergic Deficit (SWEDD). In some cases, this may be because dystonic tremor has been misdiagnosed as tremor-dominant Parkinson's disease (see pages 42–3; Table 3.2). Further long-term studies addressing the natural history of SWEDD cases are required.

Some centers employ olfactory testing using sniffin sticks or the University of Pennsylvania smell identification test (UPSIT), both of which are validated measures of olfaction. Olfaction is almost always impaired in idiopathic Parkinson's disease, but normal in essential tremor, PSP and some genetic forms of Parkinson's. In addition, it can be useful to screen for cognitive impairment, major depression and psychosis as well as RBD at an early stage of the condition.

Further investigations for young-onset or atypical disease may include the following tests at the physician's discretion:

- measurement of copper and ceruloplasmin levels, urinary copper excretion and ophthalmological examination for Kaiser–Fleischer rings to rule out Wilson's disease
- genetic tests for Huntington's disease
- tests for spinocerebellar ataxia (particularly types 3 and 17), neuroferritinopathy and other neuronal brain-iron-accumulation syndromes
- syphilis serology
- measurement of manganese levels if MRI shows increased signal in the pallidum on T1-weighted images
- genetic testing in relevant cases
- chromosome testing for fragile X syndrome, which can present with tremor and ataxia that may mimic Parkinson's disease and MSA.

In some countries such as Japan, MIBG cardiac scanning may be useful in the differential diagnosis of Parkinsonian disorders,

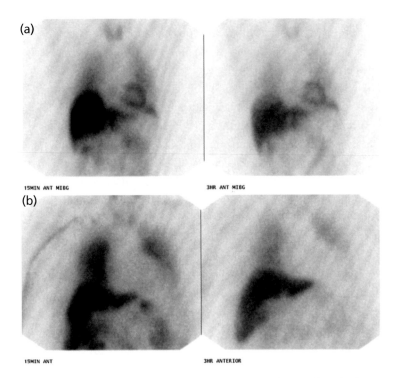

Figure 3.9 (a) Visualization of the heart 15 minutes after (left) and 3 hours after (right) intravenous injection with [^{123}I] metaiodobenzylguanidine (MIBG), showing normal activity. (b) Non-visualization of the heart 15 minutes after (left) and 3 hours after (right) intravenous injection, showing decreased cardiac MIBG activity.

particularly in the early distinction between idiopathic Parkinson's disease and atypical synucleinopathies such as MSA. Cardiac uptake measured with a MIBG scan suggests a diagnosis of atypical Parkinson's disease such as MSA, while no cardiac uptake is more suggestive of idiopathic Parkinson's disease (Figure 3.9).

Referral and 'shared care'

Current opinion and guidelines recommend that all patients with a 'suspected' diagnosis of Parkinson's disease must be referred untreated to a specialist who can reliably differentiate between Parkinson's disease and other parkinsonian syndromes. Initiation of treatment in primary care is discouraged. Referral to a specialist is important to ensure that diagnosis is as accurate as possible (approximately 96% certainty in specialist centers) and multidisciplinary team care is started promptly.

Differential diagnoses. The key differential diagnoses include essential tremor, drug-induced parkinsonism, vascular pseudoparkinsonism and the Parkinson-plus syndromes such as MSA, PSP, dementia with Lewy bodies and corticobasal ganglionic degeneration (see Chapter 8).

Key points – diagnosis

- Most cases of Parkinson's disease are recognizable at an early stage, but can be misdiagnosed if tremor is absent.
- Characteristic motor symptoms include tremor, bradykinesia, a hurried shuffling gait, freezing episodes, rigidity and a bent posture.
- Non-motor symptoms include depression, dementia, sleep disorders, bowel and bladder problems, fatigue, apathy and pain; although common, these symptoms are often overlooked.
- There are no specific tests for the diagnosis of Parkinson's disease, but DaTSCAN with single-photon emission computed tomography (SPECT) is becoming widely available, and can help to support a clinical diagnosis.
- Patients with idiopathic Parkinson's disease show a significant and sustained response to dopaminergic agents.
- Brain imaging is not typically used to diagnose Parkinson's disease, but may help to rule out tumors, vascular disease and normal-pressure hydrocephalus; transcranial ultrasound scanning reveals characteristic hyperechogenicity of the substantia nigra.
- All patients with a 'suspected' diagnosis of Parkinson's disease should be referred untreated to a specialist who can reliably differentiate between Parkinson's disease and other parkinsonian syndromes. A shared care strategy can then be implemented, with ongoing care by the primary care team.

NMSQuest scores can guide referral (i.e. the number of symptoms ticked 'yes'; see Figure 3.5); individuals with severe to very severe non-motor symptom scores have a poor quality of life irrespective of motor stage and need focused multidisciplinary care as well as management of specific non-motor symptoms.

Shared care. Once the diagnosis has been confirmed, a 'shared care' strategy should be implemented, with ongoing care undertaken by the primary care team. This is particularly important in patients with a large number of non-motor symptoms on the NMSQuest.

Key references

Albanese A, Bonuccelli U, Brefel C et al. Consensus statement on the role of acute dopaminergic challenge in Parkinson's disease. *Mov Disord* 2001;16:197–201.

Berardelli A, Wenning GK, Antonini A et al. EFNS/MDS-ES/ENS [corrected] recommendations for the diagnosis of Parkinson's disease. *Eur J Neurol* 2013;20:16–34.

Berg D, Merz B, Reiners K et al. Five-year follow-up study of hyperechogenicity of the substantia nigra in Parkinson's disease. *Mov Disord* 2005;20:383–5.

Berg D, Siefker C, Becker GJ. Echogenicity of the substantia nigra in Parkinson's disease and its relation to clinical findings. *Neurology* 2001;248:684–9.

Bötzel K, Tronnier V, Gasser T. The differential diagnosis and treatment of tremor *Dtsch Arztebl Int* 2014;111:225–35.

Chaudhuri KR, Healy DG, Schapira AH; National Institute for Health and Clinical Excellence. The non-motor symptoms of Parkinson's disease: diagnosis and management. *Lancet Neurol* 2006;5:235–45.

Chaudhuri KR, Martinez-Martin P, Brown RG et al. The metric properties of a novel non-motor symptoms scale for Parkinson's disease: results from an international pilot study. *Mov Disord* 2007;22:1901–11.

Chaudhuri KR, Martinez-Martin P, Schapira AH et al. International multicenter pilot study of the first comprehensive self-completed non-motor symptoms questionnaire for Parkinson's disease: the NMS Quest study. *Mov Disord* 2006;21:916–23.

Chaudhuri KR, Sauerbier A. Unravelling the nonmotor mysteries of Parkinson disease. *Nat Rev Neurol* 2016;12:10–11.

Chaudhuri KR, Sauerbier A, Rojo JM et al. The burden of non-motor symptoms in Parkinson's disease using a self-completed non-motor questionnaire: a simple grading system. *Parkinsonism Relat Disord* 2015;21:287–91.

Elble RJ. Defining dystonic tremor. *Curr Neuropharmacol* 2013;11: 48–52.

Fahn S, Elton RL; members of the UPDRS Development Committee. Unified Parkinson's Disease Rating Scale. In: Fahn S, Marsden CD, Calne DB, Goldstein M, eds. *Recent Developments in Parkinson's Disease,* vol 2. Florham Park, NJ: Macmillan Health Care Information, 1987:153–63, 293–304.

Ferreira JJ, Katzenschlager R, Bloem BR et al. Summary of the recommendations of the EFNS/MDS-ES review on therapeutic management of Parkinson's disease. *Eur J Neurol* 2013;20:5–15.

Hoehn MM, Yahr MD. Parkinsonism: onset, progression, and mortality. *Neurology* 1998;50:318 (reprinted from *Neurology* 1967;17:427–42).

NICE. *Parkinson's disease in over 20s: diagnosis and management. Clinical guideline 35.* London: National Institute for Health and Care Excellence, June 2006. www. nice.org.uk/guidance/cg35, last accessed 03 May 2016.

Nutt JG, Wooten GF. Clinical practice. Diagnosis and initial management of Parkinson's disease. *N Engl J Med* 2005;353:1021–7.

Olanow CW, Watts RL, Koller WC. An algorithm (decision tree) for the management of Parkinson's disease (2001): treatment guidelines. *Neurology* 2001;56(11suppl5): S1–88.

Paviour DC, Thornton JS, Lees AJ, Jager HR. Diffusion-weighted magnetic resonance imaging differentiates Parkinsonian variant of multiple-system atrophy from progressive supranuclear palsy. *Mov Disord* 2007;22:68–74.

Piccini P, Brooks DJ. New developments of brain imaging for Parkinson's disease and related disorders. *Mov Disord* 2006;21: 2035–41.

Postuma RB, Berg D, Stern M et al. MDS clinical diagnostic criteria for Parkinson's disease. *Mov Disord* 2015;30:1591–601.

Prestel J, Schweitzer KJ, Hofer A et al. Predictive value of transcranial sonography in the diagnosis of Parkinson's disease. *Mov Disord* 2006;21:1763–5.

Samii A, Nutt JG, Ransom BR. Parkinson's disease. *Lancet* 2004;363:1783–93.

Sauerbier A, Ray Chaudhuri K. Non-motor symptoms: the core of multi-morbid Parkinson's disease. *Br J Hosp Med (Lond)* 2014;75:18–24.

Zis P, Rizos A, Martinez-Martin P et al. Non-motor symptoms profile and burden in drug naïve versus long-term Parkinson's disease patients. *J Parkinsons Dis* 2014;4:541–7.

History

The first drugs used to treat Parkinson's disease, in the 1860s, were the belladonna alkaloids. These were replaced by the synthetic anticholinergic drugs benzhexol and benztropine in the 1940s, although pharmacological treatment has been the mainstay of Parkinson's disease management since the 1920s when researchers were focused on the development of a vaccine that would prevent postencephalitic parkinsonism. In 1957, Dr Arvid Carlsson demonstrated that dopamine was a neurotransmitter in the brain and not just a precursor of norepinephrine, as was the prevailing view at that time. He went on to show that L-dopa, a precursor of dopamine, effectively treated the symptoms of Parkinsonism. In 2000, he was awarded the Nobel prize for the first description of levodopa therapy in Parkinson's disease. During the 1960s, Birkmayer and Hornykiewicz, Barbeau et al. and Cotzias et al. demonstrated the dramatic clinical effects of high-dose oral levodopa therapy, revolutionizing the treatment of Parkinson's disease.

Levodopa

Levodopa is a precursor of dopamine and restores the dopamine lost due to degeneration of striatonigral cells. It has improved the quality of patients' lives substantially, and appears to have led to a reduction in mortality. Levodopa is converted to dopamine by dopa decarboxylation in the brain (Figure 4.1), but this can also occur outside the blood–brain barrier, leading to side effects such as nausea and postural hypotension. The addition of a peripheral decarboxylase inhibitor that does not cross the blood–brain barrier, such as carbidopa or benserazide, inhibits dopa decarboxylase in the rest of the body and reduces side effects. The bioavailability of levodopa has been enhanced further by the emergence of drugs such as tolcapone and entacapone, which inhibit catechol-O-methyl transferase (COMT), the enzyme principally responsible for the breakdown of dopamine.

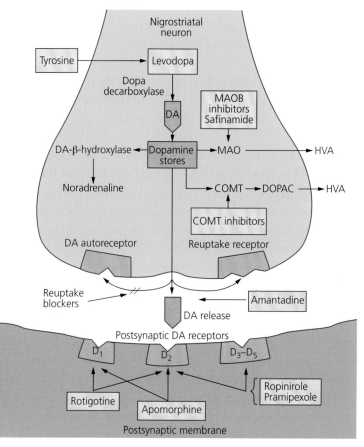

Figure 4.1 Dopamine metabolism and action of various dopaminergic drugs. COMT, catechol-O-methyl transferase; DA, dopamine; DOPAC, dihydroxyphenylacetic acid; HVA, homovanillic acid; MAO, monoamine oxidase.

Expected response. Patients with typical Parkinson's disease respond to levodopa almost immediately, although in some cases a delayed effect is seen after prolonged treatment. The beneficial response to levodopa can often be assessed after a single test dose. However, there may be significant false-positive results, given that patients with Parkinson-plus syndromes such as multiple system atrophy (MSA) or progressive supranuclear palsy (PSP) may also respond to levodopa initially. In addition, the test does not allow for the delayed positive 'long-duration' effect of levodopa. In resistant cases, the maximum

63

tolerated dose (up to 2 g/day) should be tried for at least 1 month before the patient is declared unresponsive.

Administration. Levodopa therapy should be started at the minimal effective dose (usually 50–100 mg/day), in combination with a decarboxylase inhibitor, given three times daily.

Is levodopa toxic? Results of experiments with cultured dopaminergic neurons and with rats previously suggested that levodopa may be toxic to dopamine neurons; it was postulated that levodopa is converted to toxic dopamine metabolites, which cause damage by the production of free radicals such as hydrogen peroxide. The substantia nigra was thought to be at risk because it contains high concentrations of catalysts, such as iron, for free-radical production, and low concentrations of free-radical scavengers. These concerns gave rise to 'levodopa phobia' in many patients, denying them the benefit of levodopa treatment.

However, there is no robust evidence to suggest that levodopa is toxic to the human nigrostriatal pathway and these fears have mostly been discredited. A postmortem study of 5 patients with essential tremor, who were mistakenly given sustained levodopa therapy, found no evidence of damage to nigral cells. In addition, patients who receive long-term levodopa for restless legs syndrome show no evidence of damage to the substantia nigra at autopsy. These findings should reassure patients receiving long-term levodopa.

Levodopa dyskinesia. Chronic therapy with levodopa, however, results in motor fluctuations and dyskinesias due to Parkinson's disease progression coupled with the short half-life of levodopa. The ELLDOPA study (see below) in patients with early Parkinson's disease suggests that a higher dosage of levodopa leads to a higher frequency of dyskinesia. The development of dyskinesias has been shown to adversely affect patients' and carers' quality of life, and to at least double the cost of care. In order to prevent/delay dyskinesia, several trials have examined initiating treatment with a dopamine agonist such as ropinirole, pramipexole, cabergoline or pergolide. Many trials have compared these dopamine agonists with levodopa in previously untreated patients over a 4–5 year period.

Caution is necessary when comparing results, owing to differences in the methods used, but all the studies have suggested that up to 50% fewer dyskinesias developed in those treated with a dopamine agonist rather than levodopa, which can be reserved for use when the effects of the dopamine agonist wear off.

The ELLDOPA study (Early versus Late LevoDOPA in Parkinson's disease) evaluated previously untreated patients randomized to three doses (150, 300 or 600 mg) of levodopa or placebo. Levodopa-treated patients showed a significant improvement in motor scores at all three doses compared with those receiving placebo. Single-photon emission computed tomography (SPECT) imaging suggested an increased rate of decline of striatal ^{123}I-β-CIT uptake in the levodopa-treated arm compared with placebo. This anomalous observation further deepens the confusion surrounding the use of imaging findings as surrogate markers, the link between imaging findings and clinical outcome, and whether in-vivo neuroprotection trials can really be performed.

Side effects, such as lightheadedness or nausea, may be relieved by taking medication with food or increasing the dose of decarboxylase inhibitor. Side effects usually settle but, if persistent, can be prevented by using a peripheral dopamine antagonist such as domperidone. Some complications may, however, persist in the long term (Table 4.1).

Levodopa formulations

Controlled-release preparations of levodopa, 200 mg or 100 mg, have no significant advantages over immediate-release preparations apart from their use in treating nocturnal disabilities. Such preparations have reduced bioavailability, and many patients dislike the longer lead time before improvement. Combining controlled-release and shorter-acting preparations is not advisable because the effect is difficult to predict.

Addition of a catechol-O-methyl transferase (COMT) inhibitor such as entacapone to the traditional combination of levodopa and a decarboxylase inhibitor (carbidopa) is now licensed for the treatment of later-stage Parkinson's disease that is no longer stabilized on a levodopa/decarboxylase preparation.

TABLE 4.1

Levodopa-related complications

Short term

Gastrointestinal	• Nausea, vomiting, gastritis
Cardiovascular	• Postural hypotension

Long term

Motor

Fluctuations	• 'Wearing-off' phenomenon (end-of-dose deterioration)
	• Random 'on/off' oscillations
	• Delayed 'on' response
	• Drug-resistant 'off' phenomenon (dose failure)
	• Early-morning akinesia
	• Freezing
	• Diphasic dyskinesia
Dyskinesia	• Peak-dose choreic turning 'on'

Non-motor ('off' period related)

	• Pain, akathisia, restless legs
	• Sweating, tachycardia, dyspnea
	• Depression, panic attacks, hyperventilation, screaming
	• 'Off' period dystonia
Neuropsychiatric	• Hallucinations
	• Delirium and paranoid psychosis
	• Hypersexuality
Sleep related	• Nightmares/vivid dreams
	• Fragmented sleep

The STRIDE-PD study was a prospective 134-week double-blind trial comparing the risk of developing dyskinesias in 747 Parkinson's disease patients randomized to either levodopa and carbidopa (LC) or levodopa, carbidopa and entacapone (LCE), administered four times daily at 3.5-hour intervals. LCE had a shorter time to onset and increased frequency of dyskinesia at week 134 (42% vs 32%; $p < 0.02$) than LC. The time to wearing off and motor scores were not significantly different, although there was a trend in favor of LCE.

Although the mean levodopa dose was comparable in the two groups, the LCE group had a 30% greater exposure to levodopa based on the pharmacokinetic effect of entacapone, which increases the plasma levodopa by 30%. LCE caused a significant increase in dyskinesia in patients who were taking dopamine agonists, but not in patients who were not taking dopamine agonists. Surprisingly, there was an increase in prostate cancer and myocardial infarctions in the LCE group. At present, LCE cannot be recommended as the initial levodopa formulation.

Intraduodenal/jejunal infusion of levodopa offers an alternative route of administration in very advanced Parkinson's disease when other treatments have failed, and in patients not suitable for deep brain stimulation (see Table 5.3) or apomorphine (see pages 73–4). Using a portable infusion pump the enteral gel is delivered continuously through a percutaneous endoscopic gastrostomy tube into the duodenum, where it is absorbed and produces a steady plasma level. Studies have shown that this infusion is effective in controlling motor fluctuations in advanced Parkinson's disease and reduces dyskinesias. It also enables the patient to discontinue oral dopaminergic treatment and apomorphine infusion. It is licensed in several countries as an 'orphan' drug.

Several other trials using intrajejunal levodopa are in progress or have been completed. These include the GLORIA and MONOTREAT studies (completed), and the DUOGLOBE (addressing non-motor symptoms, specifically sleep) and INSIGHTS studies (in progress).

Carbidopa/levodopa extended release. A novel extended-release capsule formulation of carbidopa and levodopa in a 1:4 ratio (ER CD-LD, formerly known as IPX066), containing intermediate- and extended-release beads, has recently been licensed for the treatment of Parkinson's disease. The drug's enhanced pharmacokinetic profile offers reliable control of motor symptoms, including the reduction of 'off time' throughout the day. Three studies have investigated the efficacy of this formulation in patients with Parkinson's disease (see below); however, no sleep benefit has been found, and the long-term consequences of this dosing with levodopa is unknown.

The APEX-PD study, a phase 3 randomized double-blind fixed-dose placebo-controlled trial, investigated the safety and efficacy of ER CD-LD in levodopa-naïve patients with early Parkinson's disease.

Patients were randomized to one of four treatments for 30 weeks: placebo or ER CD-LD, 145 mg, 245 mg or 390 mg, three times daily. All dosages were superior to placebo throughout the study and at 30 weeks ($p < 0.0001$) with respect to the change from baseline in Unified Parkinson's Disease Rating Scale (UPDRS) part II and III scores. The most frequently reported adverse events were nausea, headache and dizziness, but there were no unexpected serious adverse events related to the drug. The trial showed that ER CD-LD is safe and efficacious in patients with early Parkinson's disease.

The ADVANCE-PD study, a double-blind active-control parallel-group randomized phase 3 study, compared the efficacy and safety of ER CD-LD with immediate-release (IR) CD–LD in patients with advanced Parkinson's disease with motor fluctuations. The primary endpoint of percentage of 'off time' during waking hours showed a significant decrease for ER CD-LD compared with IR CD-LD. ER CD-LD significantly improved the control of motor symptoms compared with IR CD-LD in several clinical measures including the UPDRS, Clinician Global Impression of Change (CGI), Patient Global Impression of Change (PGI), Parkinson's Disease Questionnaire (PDQ)-39 and modified Rankin test. ER CD-LD was generally well tolerated.

The ASCEND-PD study, a randomized double-blind two-period crossover trial, compared ER CD-LD with carbidopa-levodopa in combination with the COMT inhibitor entacapone (CD-LD-E) in patients with advanced Parkinson's disease with motor fluctuations. The primary outcome measure was the percentage of 'off time' during waking hours based on subjects' diaries. ER CD-LD improved motor symptoms compared with CD-LD-E, demonstrating that it may be a useful treatment option in these patients.

Dopamine agonists

Dopamine agonists stimulate dopamine receptors directly and so bypass the degenerating presynaptic nigrostriatal neurons. Five types of dopamine receptors (D_1–D_5) have been identified so far, broadly divided into:
- D_1-like receptors (D_1 and D_5) – linked to adenylate cyclase
- D_2-like receptors (D_2, D_3 and D_4) – not linked to adenylate cyclase.

Improvement in motor function is generally attributed to D_1 and D_2 receptors, which are densely concentrated in the striatum (caudate nucleus and putamen). D_3 receptors are localized in the limbic regions that are important for regulation of behavior, mood and emotion. Ease of use, side effects and relative cost determine which dopamine agonist to choose (Table 4.2).

Efficacy. Pergolide and cabergoline are no longer recommended or in widespread use because of studies showing an association with ergot-related cardiac valvular disease. If absolutely indicated, cabergoline can only be used after pre-treatment echocardiography (ECG), with regular monitoring by ECG and chest X-ray during treatment. Lung and cardiac function should also be regularly monitored.

In this respect, non-ergot dopamine agonists such as pramipexole, ropinirole and the rotigotine transdermal patch are preferable (see Table 4.2). Longer-acting agonists such as the rotigotine skin patch, and once-daily ropinirole and pramipexole may also be used for added convenience and adherence.

Comparative studies of the efficacy of these newer dopamine agonists are scarce. The longer half-life of some dopamine agonists, and also their receptor specificity, may help in the provision of a more sustained and selective motor effect with fewer side effects (Table 4.3).

Continuous dopamine stimulation (CDS) is a relatively modern concept that has been shown to reduce the severity and incidence of dyskinesias based on the fact that pulsatile delivery of dopamine to the deafferented dopamine receptors in the striatum is likely to be dyskinesogenic.

CDS may prevent or reverse motor complications because it does not prime the basal ganglia for involuntary movements as much as agents that produce pulsatile stimulation. CDS may also improve some aspects of sleep in patients with Parkinson's disease. However, Nutt reinforced the idea that CDS remains a theoretical concept, and the effect of CDS on dyskinesias, to date, has never been tested in a robust randomized clinical trial. The STRIDE-PD study (see pages 66–7) with the drugs given orally every 3.5 hours probably failed to provide CDS.

In practice, dopamine agonists are also useful for smoothing the

TABLE 4.2

Non-ergot dopamine agonists in common use

Agonist*	Receptor selectivity	Typical dose (mg/day)[†]	Indications and advantages
Ropinirole – Rop IR – Rop XL o.d. – Adartrel (UK for RLS)	D_2+++ D_3++++	3–18 (1–24)	Adjunctive[‡] or monotherapy[§]
Pramipexole – PPX IR – PPX SR	D_2++++ D_3++++	1.5–4.5 (0.75–6)	Adjunctive[‡] or monotherapy
Rotigotine – Transdermal patch	D_1+++ D_3++	4–8[¶] (2–16)	Adjunctive or monotherapy
Apomorphine	D_1++++ D_2++++ D_3+	10–80 (3–120)	Adjunctive[‡]

*Preferably, all agonists should be used after pre-treatment with domperidone, 10 mg three times daily. Somnolence may occur with the use of all dopamine agonists, particularly in older patients (> 75 years) and at high doses. There has been increasing concern about dopamine dysregulation syndrome, punding and impulse-control disorders associated with dopaminergic treatment in individuals with a history of gambling, substance addiction and young-onset Parkinson's disease (see pages 75–7).

'on/off' fluctuations secondary to levodopa, as well as the many theoretical advantages listed in Table 4.4.

Ropinirole and pramipexole are well-established non-ergot dopamine agonists in widespread clinical use in early and advanced Parkinson's disease. Both are effective in early and late disease as monotherapy and adjunctive therapy. In addition, pramipexole has been investigated for its anti-anxiety and antidepressant effects in Parkinson's disease. A direct beneficial effect of pramipexole on depressive symptoms, accounting for 80% of total treatment effect, was found in a

Additional uses	Side effects, established/probable
RLS	Somnolence, neuropsychiatric side effects
RLS; depression	Somnolence, insomnia, neuropsychiatric side effects
Nighttime symptoms	Nausea/vomiting, skin irritation, postural hypotension
RLS; dyskinesias; pain ('off' period); dystonia; impotence	Skin nodules, postural hypotension, nausea/vomiting (preventable with domperidone)

†Values in parentheses indicate dose ranges used occasionally in clinical practice. Common dose ranges are presented without parentheses.
‡In advanced Parkinson's disease.
§Ropinirole monotherapy can be initiated with a starter and continuation pack that titrates the dose up to 9 mg/day, thus avoiding underdosing.
¶Maximum dose for monotherapy.
−, antagonist action at receptor; +, agonist action at receptor; IR, immediate release; o.d., once daily; RLS, restless legs syndrome; SR, slow release; XL, extended release.

12-week randomized double-blind placebo-controlled trial of the drug in 287 mild-to-moderate Parkinson's disease patients with depressive symptoms.

In the 1990s, 8 patients with Parkinson's disease who were taking pramipexole or ropinirole were reported to have fallen asleep while driving, causing accidents. In Europe, this led to a driving ban for patients taking either of the two drugs, although the ban has now been lifted. Since then, similar episodes of unintended sleep have been reported in patients taking other dopaminergic drugs. Daytime sleepiness is likely to be a part of the disease process, which could be

TABLE 4.3

Elimination half-lives of dopamine agonists and levodopa

Drug	Elimination half-life (hours)	Dosing regimen
Pramipexole (immediate release)	8–12	t.d.s.
Pramipexole (prolonged release)	8–12	o.d.
Ropinirole (immediate release)	6	t.d.s.
Ropinirole (prolonged release)	6	o.d.
Cabergoline	63–68	o.d.
Rotigotine (transdermal)	5–7	12–24 h/day
Lisuride	2–4	b.d. or t.d.s.
Apomorphine	0.5	s.c. 12–24 h/day
Levodopa (immediate release)	1	b.d. or t.d.s.
Levodopa (controlled release)	1.5–2	o.d. or b.d.

b.d., twice daily; o.d., once daily; s.c., subcutaneous; t.d.s., three times daily.

TABLE 4.4

Theoretical advantages of dopamine agonists

- Direct stimulation of dopamine receptors, bypassing degenerating nigrostriatal neurons
- Potential for selective dopamine receptor (D_1, D_2 or D_3) activation
- Longer striatal half-life compared with levodopa
- No intermediate step requiring enzymatic conversion to active drug
- No competition with larger neutral amino-acid transport in gut or at blood–brain barrier
- Controversial clinical evidence for possible neuroprotective disease-modifying effects
- Delayed appearance of levodopa-related side effects

aggravated by the use of dopaminergic drugs. This important side effect is discussed in greater detail on pages 136–7 (see Sleep disorders).

Rotigotine is the first transdermally delivered non-ergot dopamine agonist shown to be effective in early and advanced Parkinson's disease. Unlike the other non-ergot dopamine agonists it is effective in a once-daily application, and provides a theoretically attractive option for CDS by achieving constant plasma levels over 24 hours. In parkinsonian primate and mouse models, treatment with rotigotine produces virtually no dyskinesias.

In addition to D_3 activity, rotigotine also has considerable affinity for the D_1 receptor, unlike the other non-ergot dopamine agonists pramipexole and ropinirole. This is theoretically important because D_1 activity is thought to synergistically enhance the effect mediated via D_2-like receptors. Rotigotine appears to have no affinity for 5-HT_{2b} receptors, which have been implicated in the pathogenesis of fibrotic side effects associated with ergot dopamine agonists, particularly cardiac valvulopathy.

Transdermal delivery also offers the advantage of preventing interaction with food and the first-pass metabolism associated with oral drugs. Approximately 1200 patients were enrolled worldwide in phase 3 trials in which rotigotine provided effective relief from the symptoms of both early and advanced Parkinson's disease.

In clinical trials, a rotigotine patch was associated with a reaction at the site of application in 39–44% of patients, although only a small subset had a severe reaction. The risk is reduced by changing the application site on a daily basis.

Rotigotine patches were withdrawn from the US market because of a problem with crystallization, but were reintroduced in 2012. The licensed doses are different from those in the UK.

Apomorphine is a highly potent D_1 and D_2 agonist that also acts on D_3 receptors but has no opioid properties. It has a short half-life and is usually administered subcutaneously, either as a 'rescue' injection or by an infusion pump over 12, 18 or 24 hours. The effects of oral and rectal apomorphine are less reliable; delivery by transdermal iontophoresis, and the buccal, intranasal and rectal routes are under investigation. Occasionally, patients can stop taking levodopa, but most need regular doses in addition to apomorphine.

Apomorphine infusion benefits patients with refractory motor response fluctuations and diphasic dyskinesias. Continuous subcutaneous administration may be very useful in the later stages of the disease, producing a continuous antidyskinetic effect and smoothing 'on/off' fluctuations. In the case of injections, a response occurs after 10–15 minutes and lasts for 45–60 minutes. Self-injection, in a manner similar to the self-injection of insulin by people with diabetes, is ideal for 'rescuing' patients from disabling 'off' periods. The treatment can be labor-intensive and requires specialist nursing care. In the UK, where the treatment is well established, 'shared care' guidelines have been developed to help the delivery of apomorphine therapy, clearly setting out the shared responsibilities of primary and secondary care providers. This is not the case in the USA where apomorphine infusion is not yet licensed for use. Daily rotation of injection sites may prevent skin nodules, while local ultrasound therapy and skin massage can help to treat existing nodules.

Side effects of dopamine agonists

Nausea. The antiemetic domperidone (not available in the USA) used to be recommended for use with all dopamine agonists to prevent nausea. However, this is no longer the case as it has been found to be associated with cardiac dysrrythmia related to prologation of the QT interval. As such, the Medicines and Healthcare Products Regulatory Agency (MHRA) has advised that domperidone, 10 mg three times daily, should only be used for a maximum of 1 week. In the USA, alternative antiemetics such as trimethobenzamide, 250 mg three times daily, are used in conjunction with apomorphine to prevent nausea.

Sleep disorders. Unintended or abnormal sleepiness is a potentially dangerous adverse effect in patients taking dopaminergic agents. As well as the incidents reported in patients taking ropinirole and pramipexole (see page 71), similar episodes have been reported in patients taking pergolide, bromocriptine, cabergoline, apomorphine and levodopa. However, abnormal sleepiness has also been described in patients with Parkinson's disease at the time of diagnosis, when they are not yet receiving any dopamine-replacement therapy. Daytime sleepiness is, therefore, likely to be a combined effect of the disease process and dopaminergic drug treatment, and not a novel event related solely to the use of dopamine agonists.

A small percentage of patients with Parkinson's disease (possibly 0.5–1%) with excessive daytime sleepiness, may exhibit sudden onset of sleep resembling narcolepsy. For this reason, older patients receiving dopaminergic therapy should be assessed using both the Epworth Sleepiness Scale (for excessive daytime sleepiness) and the Parkinson's Disease Sleep Scale (PDSS). A pragmatic view is that those who score more than 10 out of 24 on the Epworth scale, or less than 5 on item 15 of the PDSS, should be advised to exercise caution when driving, or preferably not to drive at all during the titration phase of therapy.

Studies suggest that somnolence is at its worst when dopaminergic therapy, particularly treatment with dopamine agonists, is being initiated and titrated up. In 'sleepy' patients, polysomnography may identify a subset of people with a phenotype similar to that for narcolepsy, or it may unearth sleep apnea as a cause of daytime sleepiness.

Dopamine dysregulation syndrome (DDS), which resembles addiction, has been described in mostly young male patients with Parkinson's disease. DDS is typically linked to levodopa therapy when doses are increased continuously and beyond the level required to treat motor disability. The emerging pattern is that of a compulsive medication overuse associated with cognitive and behavioral disturbances. Patients are also liable to develop impulse-control disorders or punding behavior. Patients crave the drug and have unpleasant 'off' periods. As a result, they increase the dose of drugs that have been prescribed 'as required' or increase doses for reported 'off' periods. Patients often seek alternative drug sources such as internet sites, and drug hoarding and hiding are common. The condition has been termed variously as:
- homeostatic hedonistic dysregulation
- impulse dysregulation
- compulsive behavior syndrome
- reward-seeking behavior.

Punding may be seen in association with DDS or in isolation, and implies an intense fascination with repetitive tasks. These complex repetitive behaviors were first described in psychostimulant addicts, and the phenomenon is similar to that observed in animals with amphetamine-induced stereotyped behaviors. The behaviors may develop from pre-existing habits, depending on an individual's previous occupation and interests. Examples include hoarding, handling, labeling and sorting objects, spending excessive time on a computer, writing or drawing, and aimless walkabouts. In men, the manipulation or dismantling of machines and tools is often reported.

Impulse-control disorders. The American Psychiatric Association's DSM5 (*Diagnostic and Statistical Manual of Mental Disorders*, 5th edition) defines impulse control disorders (ICDs) as the failure to resist an impulse, drive or temptation to perform an act that is harmful to the person or to others. These are increasingly reported in Parkinson's disease and include a range of compulsive disorders (Table 4.5).

TABLE 4.5

Impulse control disorders associated with Parkinson's disease

- Pathological gambling
- Compulsive sexual behaviors
  - hypersexuality including paraphilias
  - disinhibition
  - addiction to pornography
- Compulsive internet use
- Binge eating/compulsive eating/night eating
- Hobbyism
- Reckless generosity
- Compulsive shopping/excessive spending
- Kleptomania
- Pyromania
- Walkabout

Typically, the syndrome is characterized by a combination of impulsivity, compulsivity and preoccupation with a behavior or mood state. Unrecognized, ICDs can have serious consequences, such as breakdowns in interpersonal relationships and financial distress. The lifetime prevalence of ICDs, as reported by patients attending specialized clinics, is between 3 and 8%, although the DOMINION study reported a higher rate of 13.7% with ICDs, including problem/pathological gambling (5%), compulsive sexual behavior (3.5%), compulsive buying (5.7%) and binge-eating disorder (4.3%).

Men with early-onset Parkinson's disease and a history of alcohol misuse, illicit drug use or affective disorders may be susceptible to this syndrome. Abnormal dopamine release in the nucleus accumbens in response to a reward has been postulated as a possible mechanism. The treatment is complex and requires slow withdrawal of dopamine agonists, use of atypical neuroleptics and/or antidepressants, counseling and input from a neuropsychiatrist.

Dopamine agonist withdrawal syndrome. Abrupt cessation of therapy with dopamine agonists can lead to a dopamine agonist withdrawal syndrome (DAWS). It can present with a wide range of symptoms including panic attacks, anxiety, social phobia, depression, vomiting and symptomatic orthostatic hypotension. It rarely responds to levodopa, antidepressants or anxiolytics. However, it may improve with cautious reintroduction of low-dose dopamine agonists.

Fibrosis. The risk of serosal fibrosis in relation to ergot-derived drugs was first described in 1966. There have been several reports of cardiac, retroperitoneal and pleuropulmonary fibrosis in patients taking ergot-derived dopamine agonists such as pergolide, cabergoline and bromocriptine. Serosal fibrosis is a serious complication that is often irreversible.

The increased affinity of ergot-derived dopamine agonists for 5-HT_{2b} receptors has been cited as a possible mechanism. In practice, given the availability of non-ergot agonists (see above), the use of ergot dopamine agonists is no longer recommended.

Catechol-*O*-methyl transferase inhibitors

COMT metabolizes dopamine and levodopa, producing two inactive metabolites, 3-O-methyl-dopamine and 3-O-methyl-dopa. Two COMT inhibitors, tolcapone and entacapone, are available; they extend the plasma half-life of levodopa, thus increasing the concentrations of levodopa and dopamine within the brain (Table 4.6; Figure 4.2). COMT inhibition prolongs 'on' time by 30–60%, which may increase the duration of, but not worsen, peak-dose dyskinesias.

Tolcapone blocks COMT in both the peripheral and central nervous systems. In November 1998, the European Medical Evaluation Agency withdrew tolcapone in the EU because of three cases of fatal fulminant hepatitis; sales were also suspended in Canada and Australia. In the USA, the Food and Drug Administration (FDA) recommended that regular liver function tests be performed. Tolcapone was re-released in Europe, but now its use must be accompanied by regular blood tests to monitor liver function. The FDA advises that levels of alanine and aspartate transaminase (ALT/AST) should be determined at baseline, then every 2–4 weeks during the first 6 months of therapy and then at intervals deemed clinically relevant. In the USA, tolcapone should be discontinued if ALT or AST levels exceed two times the normal upper limit. The patient consent form has been replaced with a patient acknowledgment form. The usual starting dose is 100 mg/day, increasing

TABLE 4.6

Catechol-*O*-methyl transferase inhibitors in Parkinson's disease

- *Never* use entacapone without levodopa
- Tolcapone should be used with regular liver function tests only
- Useful for early or moderately advanced disease with motor fluctuations and 'wearing off'
- Reduce levodopa dose by about 20% in dyskinetic patients, as use may worsen diphasic dyskinesia
- Entacapone and tolcapone may color urine reddish-orange
- Sudden withdrawal may cause an akinetic crisis

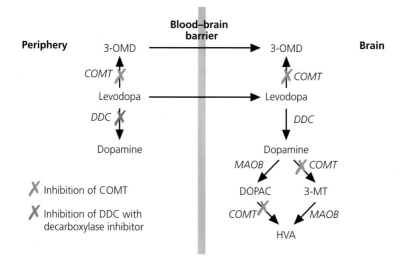

Figure 4.2 The mechanism of catechol-*O*-methyl transferase (COMT) inhibition. DDC, dopa decarboxylase; DOPAC, dihydroxyphenylacetic acid; HVA, homovanillic acid; MAOB, monoamine oxidase B; 3-MT, 3-methoxytyramine; 3-OMD, 3-*O*-methyl-dopa.

to 200 mg three times daily. Dyskinesia and nausea are common side effects, but diarrhea is the most common reason for drug withdrawal. Patients should be warned that the drug may color their urine.

Entacapone, 200 mg with each dose of levodopa, acts only peripherally, unlike tolcapone. No hepatobiliary side effects have been reported, and routine liver function tests are not required. The incidence of diarrhea is also less frequent than with tolcapone. Other side effects include hypotension, sedation, headache and dyskinesias. Patients should be forewarned that the drug may turn urine a reddish-orange color.

A combined formulation of entacapone, decarboxylase inhibitor and levodopa has been licensed for use in the USA, Europe and certain parts of Asia; the drug should make adherence easier for patients taking entacapone and is likely to be administered for treatment of early 'wearing-off' symptoms. Its use may be refined with a new scale/ questionnaire designed to assess 'wearing off', as described by Stacy et al.

Monoamine oxidase B inhibitors

Selegiline, 10 mg once daily or 5 mg twice daily orally (or 1.25 mg once daily by buccal administration), is a selective irreversible blocker of intra- and extraneuronal MAOB, and reduces metabolism of dopamine (Figure 4.3). The sublingual form of selegiline (1.25–2.5 mg/day) can be administered as an adjunct to levodopa in patients with fluctuations.

In animal models, selegiline blocks the conversion of MPTP to MPP$^+$, which is toxic to dopaminergic neurons (see Figure 2.4). On this basis, it was thought that MAOB inhibition with selegiline might slow the decline in human Parkinson's disease by neuroprotection. However, the double-blind prospective placebo-controlled DATATOP study (Deprenyl And Tocopherol Antioxidant Therapy for Parkinsonism) in 1993, failed to confirm the neuroprotective property of selegiline. Furthermore, in the mid-1990s a report by the Parkinson's Disease Research Group (UK) suggested a 60% increase in mortality among patients receiving continued selegiline therapy, although this has not been substantiated.

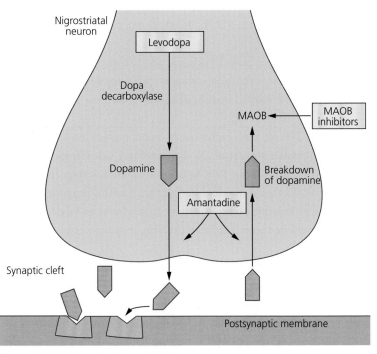

Figure 4.3 Action of presynaptic drugs.

TABLE 4.7

Monoamine oxidase inhibitors in Parkinson's disease

- May be given on its own in early stage of Parkinson's disease or in combination with other drugs
- Prolong the efficacy of dopamine
- Reduce the required amount of levodopa
- Useful for reducing fluctuations
- Should avoid in combination with antidepressants that increase the serotonin level (CAVE serotonin syndrome)

Side effects of MAOB inhibition include hallucinations, sleep disorders, agitation, postural hypotension and withdrawal problems. Although a lower-dose formulation of selegiline (2.5 mg) with a better safety profile is available, its clinical role remains unclear: it is not neuroprotective, and safety in older patients is uncertain. However, it can have a useful dopa-sparing effect and may stimulate drowsy patients (Table 4.7).

Rasagiline is a second-generation irreversible selective MAOB inhibitor that is administered orally at a dosage of 0.5–1 mg once daily. Approved dosing of this drug varies in different countries: the approved dose in Europe is 1 mg, while both 0.5 mg and 1 mg doses are approved in the USA, so that adjunctive therapy initiated at 0.5 mg can be raised to 1 mg if effectiveness is insufficient at the lower dose. It is approximately five times more potent than selegiline, and, in animal models, rasagiline increased cellular antioxidant activity and antiapoptotic factors.

In clinical trials, patients started late on rasagiline appeared to have worse motor scores than those initiated on rasagiline, prompting some researchers to suggest that rasagiline may have a disease-modifying role in Parkinson's disease (see Neuroprotection, pages 89–91). Several randomized controlled trials have shown rasagiline's efficacy as monotherapy or as an adjunct to levodopa in Parkinson's disease.

Safinamide is a glutamate antagonist as well as a MAOB inhibitor and a partial dopamine agonist. Trials suggest that this agent may improve motor function and reduce dyskinesias in patients with Parkinson's

81

disease, and may have some additional non-motor benefits. Safinamide has been approved in the EU (but is not yet licensed in the UK) as oral once-daily add-on therapy to levodopa alone or in combination with other treatments in patients with mid- to late-stage Parkinson's disease.

Phase 3 trials have shown that safinamide significantly improves motor function in early Parkinson's disease in patients taking a single dopamine agonist at a stable dose (MOTION study) and significantly improves motor fluctuations in patients with mid- to late-stage disease taking levodopa and other Parkinson's disease drugs at a stable dose (SETTLE study). Safinamide has also demonstrated statistically significant improvement in quality of life in the short (6 months) and long term (up to 2 years), as assessed by the Parkinson's Disease Quality of Life (PDQ-39) and/or the European Quality of Life (EuroQoL, EQ-5D) scales.

Anticholinergics

Anticholinergics block the action of acetylcholine against dopamine within the basal ganglia (Figure 4.4). Data on the comparative efficacies of the different anticholinergic drugs are not available.

Historically, these drugs were used as an adjunct to levodopa therapy, helping to control rest-tremor and dystonia. However, they are no longer recommended in modern practice, particularly in older parkinsonian patients because of the risk of inducing a confusional state and aggravating/accelerating dementia.

Side effects include urinary retention, constipation, blurred vision, precipitation of narrow-angle glaucoma, dry mouth, memory problems and confusion. If neuropsychiatric side effects necessitate withdrawal of anticholinergic therapy, this should be carried out slowly in order to avoid a withdrawal syndrome that itself includes a confusional state associated with akinesia and disorientation.

Other drugs

Pardoprunox is a partial dopamine agonist (mainly at D_2 and D_3 receptors) and also a full 5-HT_{1A} receptor agonist. It is being investigated for use in levodopa-treated fluctuating patients and its effect on 'off' and 'on' times without troublesome dyskinesias.

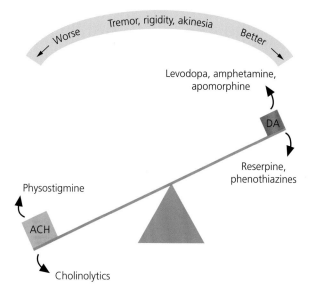

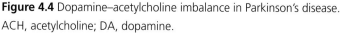

Figure 4.4 Dopamine–acetylcholine imbalance in Parkinson's disease. ACH, acetylcholine; DA, dopamine.

Amantadine, 100–400 mg daily, is an antiviral agent with an antiparkinsonian effect. Its mechanisms of action include:
- increased dopamine synthesis
- an amphetamine-like action releasing catecholamines from presynaptic stores
- blocking dopamine and noradrenaline reuptake
- mild anticholinergic action
- antiglutamate action by antagonism at the N-methyl-D-aspartate receptors.

The antiparkinsonian effect of amantadine is mild, and is useful in young patients to delay the introduction of levodopa. The effect is long-lasting, and patients may deteriorate markedly if the drug is withdrawn.

Amantadine should be given as a single dose in the morning to prevent sleep problems. At high doses, amantadine has an antidyskinetic action that may last up to 9 months, but high doses can cause visual hallucinations, confusion and agitation. Amantadine can cause a specific discoloration of the legs called livedo reticularis.

TABLE 4.8

Factors to consider when starting treatment

- Involvement of dominant hand relative to non-dominant hand
- Effect on employment/occupation
- The particular subtype of Parkinson's disease (bradykinesia-dominant disease may require earlier treatment than tremor-dominant disease)
- The individual sentiments of patients and carers (offer informed choice)
- NMSQuest-based assessment* (high non-motor scores may influence early treatment)

NMSQuest, Non-Motor Symptom Questionnaire. *NMSQuest grading helps to establish the burden of non-motor symptoms. See Figure 3.6 for an explanation of NMSQuest scores.

When to initiate treatment

Precisely when to begin treatment is controversial (Table 4.8). Some experts advocate early treatment to provide maximum clinical benefit to patients, whereas others prefer to delay initiation of treatment in order to minimize the risk of medication-related side effects including levodopa-related motor complications. The misconception that the benefits of levodopa treatment are limited to a finite period of time has caused many physicians to inappropriately delay the introduction of symptomatic therapy. With the development of pharmaceutical agents that are safe and well tolerated, with the potential to influence disease outcomes, there has been a call to reconsider the potential value of early intervention.

PDLIFE study. The argument for treatment of Parkinson's disease at diagnosis has been strengthened by the publication of the UK's prospective PDLIFE study, a national audit of the quality of life of people with Parkinson's disease. Findings indicate a progressive and significant deterioration in the self-reported health status of patients with Parkinson's disease who are left untreated at diagnosis compared with those who are treated. The work has reignited the debate of whether to initiate treatment of the disease at diagnosis or whether to adopt a 'wait and watch' policy. If a neuroprotective agent became available it would be instituted as early as possible, even before the appearance of motor symptoms. Nevertheless, the issue of neuroprotection in Parkinson's disease remains controversial (see pages 89–92).

Choice of treatment

All patients with Parkinson's disease who require drug treatment should be given the opportunity to make an informed choice from the range of treatment options available, including dopamine agonists, other levodopa-sparing agents, levodopa and combination therapy. The main aims are to:

- keep the drug regimen as simple as possible
- aid adherence
- reduce the likelihood of side effects.

Theoretically, attempts should be made to stick to a regimen that mimics CDS as much as possible. Long-acting agents, or continuous delivery systems such as the rotigotine transdermal patch, or controlled-release preparations of other non-ergot dopamine agonists may be particularly useful in this regard.

It is very important that the patient's lifestyle, amount of support at home and individual preferences are all taken into consideration, and that the different therapeutic options with their potential side effects and advantages are explained.

Modern management of Parkinson's disease is not possible without the support of a multidisciplinary care team. A typical multidisciplinary team should consist of a Parkinson's disease nurse specialist, a physiotherapist, occupational therapist, and an experienced speech and language therapist with access to neuropsychology and palliative care.

Current guidelines. Different international guidelines (NICE, AAN, EFNS/MDS-ES) all agree that there is no single universal first choice of drug for people with Parkinson's disease, particularly in the early stages of the condition. Individual choice of drug will be influenced, for example, by the degree of motor disability (if severe, the first choice is likely to be levodopa), occupational needs, the risk of motor complications (more common in younger patients, which would be delayed by agonists), neuropsychiatric complications (more common in older and cognitively impaired patients, so agonists should be avoided), patient/clinician preferences and adherence issues. For these reasons, many younger patients will choose a levodopa-sparing strategy, while older patients may prefer levodopa therapy (see below).

Guidelines for the management of Parkinson's disease published in the UK by NICE in June 2006 offer evidence-based advice drawn up by a multidisciplinary panel. Key recommendations are that patients and their carers should be involved in deciding their treatment and care, and that the choice of treatment should suit the patient's needs and preferences. This guideline is currently being updated. The following key points were identified as priorities for implementation.

- Any patient with a suspected diagnosis of Parkinson's disease should be seen by a specialist within 6 weeks after referral by the primary care physician. A specialist is defined as an individual with expertise in the differential diagnosis of Parkinson's disease.
- The diagnosis of Parkinson's disease should be reviewed every 6–12 months. The apomorphine and levodopa challenge tests should not be used to differentiate Parkinson's disease from atypical parkinsonian syndromes.
- Regular access to specialist nursing care, physiotherapy, occupational therapy, and speech and language therapy should be available to patients.
- Patients and their carers should be given an opportunity to discuss palliative care issues. No specific agents could be identified as the treatment of choice in either early or advanced disease.

The guidelines also emphasize the need for considering non-motor symptoms at all stages of Parkinson's disease.

Guidelines for the management of Parkinson's disease in other countries are broadly similar to the NICE guidelines. They include those of the AAN, published in 2002 and modified in 2006, and those issued by the joint task force of the EFNS and the Movement Disorder Society's European Section in 2006.

More recent guidelines from the Scottish Intercollegiate Guidelines Network (SIGN) highlight the following issues as key to the modern 'holistic' treatment of Parkinson's disease:

- communication throughout disease progression
- attitudes to drug treatment
- information needs in relation to multifaceted areas
- family carers' needs
- non-motor symptoms
- importance of multidisciplinary team working.

The SIGN's suggested scheme for therapy is shown in Figure 4.5.

Dopamine agonist versus levodopa. In younger patients, the issues of neuroprotection and dyskinesias should be considered. The results of four controlled dopamine-agonist monotherapy trials have been published and suggest that initiation of treatment with an agonist is

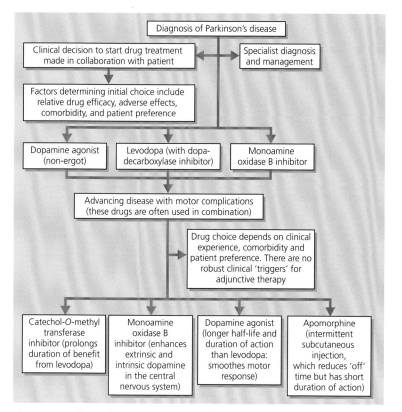

Figure 4.5 Scheme for treatment of Parkinson's disease from the Scottish Intercollegiate Guidelines Network (2010).

beneficial in the early stages of Parkinson's disease. However, the results of the PD Med study, a multicenter real-life pragmatic study, reporting on quality of life-related outcomes in both young and old patients with Parkinson's disease, is likely to generate considerable controversy regarding the use of dopamine agonists and the choice of initial therapy. In total, 1620 patients with early Parkinson's disease were recruited and given one of three initial treatment regimens:

- levodopa formulation (528 patients)
- levodopa-sparing strategy – dopamine agonist (632 patients)
- levodopa-sparing strategy – MAOB inhibitor (selegiline; 460 patients).

The study started in 2000 with a median follow-up of 3 years and maximum of 7 years. During this time the dopamine agonists varied, including ergot agonists that are no longer in widespread use. The randomization to levodopa or alternative regimens was at the discretion of the clinician and a large part of the study was conducted in centers for the care of the elderly. The findings suggest relatively small but persistent benefits of starting therapy with levodopa rather than the listed alternatives. Interestingly, initial treatment with a MAOB inhibitor appeared to be at least as effective as treatment with a dopamine agonist.

Patients assigned to the levodopa arm scored, on average, 1.8 points (95% CI 0.5–3.0) higher on the Parkinson's Disease Questionnaire-39 (PDQ-39) mobility subscale than those assigned to levodopa-sparing therapies; however, the effects on non-motor aspects of the scale are unclear. A cost-utility analysis of the study will be reported separately.

If levodopa is used and the dose is titrated to the response, most patients initially need 50–100 mg three times daily to produce a consistent effect without fluctuations. Within 2–3 years, most will need a more frequent dosage to avoid fluctuations; smaller, more frequent doses (every 2–3 hours) often lead to an overall increase in dose. COMT inhibitors or dopamine agonists can, however, be introduced instead of increasing the frequency of levodopa.

Monitoring. Scales for monitoring Parkinson's disease, and thus the response to treatment, include:

- Movement Disorder Society's UPDRS
- Hoehn and Yahr Disease Staging Scale (Table 4.9)

TABLE 4.9

The Hoehn and Yahr classification of Parkinson's disease

Stage	Characteristics
0	No signs of disease
1	Unilateral involvement only; minimal or no functional impairment
1.5	Unilateral disease, plus axial involvement
2	Bilateral disease, without impairment of balance
2.5	Mild bilateral disease with recovery on pull test
3	Mild to moderate bilateral disease; some postural instability; physically independent
4	Severe disability; still able to walk or stand unassisted
5	Wheelchair bound or bedridden unless aided

- Parkinson's Disease Questionnaire (long form – PDQ 39; short form – PDQ 8)
- EuroQol (patient-related quality of life)
- Carer Strain Index
- Epworth Sleepiness Scale
- Parkinson's Disease Sleep Scale
- Non-Motor Symptoms Questionnaire (NMSQuest; see Figure 3.5)
- Non-Motor Symptoms Scale (NMSS)
- Parkinson's Disease Fatigue Scale.

Neuroprotection

Neuroprotection is a concept whereby a treatment may affect the underlying pathophysiology of Parkinson's disease and slow or halt the inexorable progression of the condition. Neuroprotective therapies already investigated or under review include caffeine, minocycline, nicotine, estrogen, creatine, lazaroids, bioenergetics, antiapoptotic drugs (CEP-1347, TCH-346), GM-1 ganglioside and GPi-1485. MAOB inhibitors and dopamine agonists have been clinically evaluated for neuroprotective properties based on positive results in animal models.

In the early 2000s, the CALM-PD study (Comparison of the Agonist pramipexole vs Levodopa on Motor complications in Parkinson's Disease) and the REAL-PET study (Ropinirole as EArly therapy versus Levodopa – PET study) generated speculation among researchers that dopamine agonists such as ropinirole and pramipexole may have a neuroprotective role. The results were reported as partially positive, although methodological and logistical problems with these studies have prevented recommendation of these drugs specifically for neuroprotection. The trial designs did not take non-motor symptoms into account and could not exclude the regulatory effect of drugs on the imaging findings. Furthermore, clinical rating scales showed that the patients who received levodopa had better outcomes than those who received the agonists.

Trials with CEP-1347 and TCH-346, and more recently smilagenin, have been negative. Coenzyme Q10 has demonstrated encouraging potential as a neuroprotective agent in large doses, but trial data have been negative. In the USA, small 'futility studies' are being supported by the National Institute of Neurological Disorders and Stroke (NINDS) and the Michael J Fox Foundation to investigate agents with the potential to slow progression of the disease. See Chapter 9 (pages 155–8) for more information on emerging therapies in this area.

The ADAGIO study. Rasagiline has been studied in the delayed-start ADAGIO study (Attenuation of Disease progression with Azilect Once-daily), which comprised two phases, each lasting 36 weeks. In phase 1, patients were randomized to one of four groups: rasagiline, 1 mg or 2 mg/day (early-start group), or corresponding placebo. In phase 2, the subjects in the early-start group remained on the same regimen, while the subjects in the placebo group were switched to rasagiline 1 mg or 2 mg/day (delayed-start group). At the end of the study, the early-start group who had received rasagiline 1 mg/day for 72 weeks showed a positive result, but those who had received 2 mg/day for the full study period did not. The reasons for this discrepancy are unclear but may be partly explained by a more robust symptomatic benefit from the 2 mg dose that masked the disease-modifying effect. Post hoc subgroup analysis showed a positive result for both the 1 mg and 2 mg dose for those subjects who had the highest quartile scores on the UPDRS at baseline. Although this does not make the study positive, it does suggest the need for further research, i.e. larger and longer delayed-start studies using the 2 mg/day dose in patients with more advanced Parkinson's disease.

It should be noted that the difference in UPDRS between the early- and delayed-start groups was small (1.7 points) and its clinical significance is hard to ascertain. However, the object of this study was not to determine the clinical significance of a disease-modifying therapy, but to see if the benefit from therapy was secondary to disease modification, i.e. something more than symptomatic improvement.

The ADAGIO study is an important landmark clinical trial that suggests early treatment with rasagiline, 1 mg/day, confers benefits that are not duplicated by delayed treatment with the same agent. However, no 'definitive' recommendations or guidelines can be made from these results. Clinicians will have to decide on a case-by-case basis whether the patient would benefit from rasagiline. Cost, concomitant medications and a possible disease-modifying benefit will have to be factored into the decision-making process by the patient and the treating physician.

The ADAGIO Follow-Up (AFU) study investigated the long-term effect of rasagiline in ADAGIO study participants and the long-term benefits of early- versus delayed-start rasagiline treatment. Although clinically important improvements were seen in a substantial number of patients, the study failed to demonstrate significant differences between the original ADAGIO early- and delayed-start groups. However, these results should be interpreted with caution given the significant gap, and loss of participants, between the time of the ADAGIO and AFU studies.

The PROUD study (PRamipexole On Underlying Disease) is another delayed-start trial, which investigated the disease-modifying effect of pramipexole in early Parkinson's disease. In phase 1, 535 patients were randomized to double-blind placebo or pramipexole, 1.5 mg/day for 6–9 months. In phase 2, all patients were administered pramipexole, 1.5 mg/day, for up to 15 months. The primary endpoint was a change from the baseline UPDRS total score after 15 months, and a substudy assessed the change in DaTSCAN uptake after

15 months. In total, 411 patients were included in the primary assessment. After 15 months there was no difference between the early- and delayed-start group and DaTSCAN uptake was also similar. The results did not support a disease-modifying effect of pramipexole.

Treatment of non-motor symptoms

The AAN and MDS task force documents for managing non-motor symptoms of Parkinson's disease recognize the need for clinical studies in this area, as good quality trials providing a level 1 evidence base for the treatment of non-motor symptoms are few and far between. Table 4.10 summarizes the evidence base for the treatment of the small number of non-motor symptoms for which controlled trials have been conducted. The few randomized controlled studies that have addressed the non-motor aspects of Parkinson's disease are outlined below.

The RECOVER study (Randomized Evaluation of the 24-hour COVerage: Efficacy of Rotigotine) was a multinational double-blind placebo-controlled trial of 287 patients with Parkinson's disease who had unsatisfactory early-morning symptom control. Patients received either a rotigotine transdermal patch, 2–16 mg/day (n = 190), or placebo (n = 97). This was the first time an international clinical trial protocol included measures of non-motor symptoms, such as nocturnal sleep disturbance, along with early morning motor function as co-primary efficacy endpoints using the UPDRS Part III (motor examination) and the modified Parkinson's Disease Sleep Scale (PDSS-2). The overall effect on non-motor symptoms was also assessed using the Parkinson's disease non-motor scale (NMSS).

As well as significant motor improvement with rotigotine patch therapy ($p = 0.0002$), there was highly significant improvement in the mean PDSS-2 total score (a decrease of –5.9 points with rotigotine vs –1.9 points with placebo, $p < 0.0001$). The NMSS score also registered a significant improvement in sleep and mood.

Detailed post hoc analysis of the RECOVER data has shown efficacy for mild to moderate pain in Parkinson's disease as well as sleep and mood. The rotigotine transdermal patch is now being investigated for pain in Parkinson's disease using the King's Parkinson disease pain scale.

TABLE 4.10

Evidence base for the treatment of non-motor symptoms in Parkinson's disease*

- Sexual dysfunction
  - Sildenafil citrate, 50 mg (PD with ED; level C)
- Constipation
  - Isomotic macrogol (polyethylene glycol; level C)
- Sialorrhea and dribbling of saliva
  - Botulinum toxin injection (level B)
- Excessive daytime sleepiness
  - Modafinil (for patients to improve their subjective perception of EDS; level A)
- RLS/PLMS
  - Levodopa/carbidopa should be considered to treat PLMS (level B)
  - There is insufficient evidence to support or refute the treatment of RLS and PLMS with non-ergot dopamine agonists (level U)
- Fatigue
  - Methylphenidate may be considered in patients with fatigue (level C)
  - Potential for abuse

*Report of the Quality Standards Subcommittee of the American Academy of Neurology.
Level A, established as effective, ineffective or harmful; Level B, probably effective, ineffective or harmful; Level C, possibly effective, ineffective or harmful; Level U, data inadequate or conflicting.
ED, erectile dysfunction; EDS, excessive daytime sleepiness; PD, Parkinson's disease; PLMS, periodic limb movements of sleep; RLS, restless legs syndrome.

PANDA was a multisite double-blind randomized placebo-controlled parallel-group study in male and female subjects with confirmed Parkinson's disease and severe pain, as assessed by a new pain classification system for Parkinson's disease. The study evaluated treatment with prolonged-release oxycodone combined with naloxone (OXN PR). Subjects were randomized to receive either OXN PR or placebo for up to 112 days. The primary endpoint of improvement of average 24-hour pain score after 16 weeks was not met in the full analysis population but the per protocol population analysis revealed that adherence to OXN PR significantly improved average 24-hour pain scores at 16 weeks compared with placebo (p = 0.010). Furthermore, the results showed a significant improvement in the 24-hour pain score after 4 weeks (p = 0.018), 8 weeks (p = 0.011) and 12 weeks (p = 0.021). This was the first ever randomized placebo-controlled study to assess Parkinson's-associated pain as a primary outcome measure.

The EuroInf study, an open-label prospective observational 6-month multicenter study, compared 43 patients on apomorphine with 44 on intrajejunal levodopa infusion (IJLI). It is the first study to consider non-motor symptom scores as the primary outcome. Patients treated with IJLI showed large improvement (effect size = 0.83) on the NMSS total score. Patients treated with apomorphine had moderate improvement (effect size = 0.53) on the NMSS total score with significantly more improvement in mood and apathy NMSS scores than IJLI.

Overall, health-related quality of life and non-motor symptoms improved in 75% of patients receiving IJLI; a similar proportion of patients receiving apomorphine showed improvement in health-related quality of life. Adverse effects included peritonitis with IJLI and skin nodules with apomorphine.

The IMPACT study, a non-randomized controlled trial, was conducted in six hospitals in the Netherlands to address the role of a multidisciplinary approach for the treatment of Parkinson's disease. The primary outcomes were activities of daily living measured with the Academic Medical Center linear disability score and quality of life measured with the Parkinson's disease quality of life questionnaire. Results were analysed at 4, 6 and 8 months. Secondary outcomes included motor functioning (measured by UPDRS part III at 4 months), and caregiver burden and costs (during the whole study period). The results showed that the multidisciplinary care approach conferred only small benefits compared with normal integrated care in the Netherlands. The study did not reach statistical significance. However, the authors concluded that alternative approaches need to be devised and explored to achieve more substantial health benefits.

Key points – drug treatment

- Levodopa restores the dopamine lost due to degeneration of striatonigral cells; patients with typical Parkinson's disease respond to levodopa almost immediately.
- Fear over the toxicity of levodopa has resulted in levodopa phobia in some patients; however, there is no robust evidence to suggest that levodopa is toxic to the human nigrostriatal pathway and these fears have mostly been discredited.
- Dopamine agonists are useful for smoothing the 'on/off' fluctuations secondary to levodopa therapy; some, such as rotigotine, may offer continuous dopaminergic stimulation in practice and specifically offer night-time and early morning benefit.
- Treatment decisions should be based on the degree of disability, occupational needs, age, patient/clinician preference and adherence issues; neuroprotection remains a theoretical argument, while dyskinesias and wearing off are an important consideration in younger patients.
- Trial data indicate that treatment of Parkinson's disease could be initiated with levodopa, oral dopamine agonists or a monoamine oxidase B (MAOB) inhibitor. The PD MED study seems to suggest that initial therapy with levodopa offers a small but persistent benefit compared with the alternatives, and initial MAOB inhibitor treatment is at least as effective as a dopamine agonist.
- The findings of the PDLIFE study suggest that early initiation of treatment may be beneficial in terms of health-related quality of life.
- Impuse control disorders have emerged as a major complication of mostly dopamine agonist treatment, and monitoring is a must.
- The treatment of non-motor symptoms is important at all stages of Parkinson's disease. The results of the PANDA study may help people with Parkinson's-associated pain.

Key references

Albin RL, Frey KA. Initial agonist treatment of Parkinson's disease: a critique. *Neurology* 2003;60:390–4.

Barbeau A, Sourkes TL, Murphy GF. J Ajuriaguerra (ed). Les catecholamines dans la maladie de Parkinson. In: *Monoamines et système nerveux central*. Paris: Masson, 1962:247–62.

Barone P, Poewe W, Albrecht S et al. Pramipexole for the treatment of depressive symptoms in patients with Parkinson's disease: a randomised, double-blind, placebo-controlled trial. *Lancet Neurol* 2010;9:573–80.

Birkmayer W, Hornykiewicz O. Der l-Dioxyphenylalanin (=DOPA) Effekt beim Parkinson-Syndrom des Menschen: Zur Pathogenese und Behandlung der Parkinson-Akinese. *Arch Psychiatr Nervenkr* 1962;203: 560–74.

Chaudhuri KR, Pal S, Brefel-Courbon C. 'Sleep attacks' or 'unintended sleep episodes' occur with dopamine agonists: is this a class effect? *Drug Saf* 2002;25:473–83.

Cotzias GC, Van Woert MH, Schiffer LM. Aromatic amino acids and modification of parkinsonism. *N Engl J Med* 1967;276:374–9.

Dhawan V, Healy DG, Pal S, Chaudhuri KR. Sleep-related problems of Parkinson's disease. *Age Ageing* 2006;35:220–8.

Ferreira JJ, Katzenschlager R, Bloem BR et al. Summary of the recommendations of the EFNS/MDS-ES review on therapeutic management of Parkinson's disease. *Eur J Neurol* 2013;20:5–15.

Fudalej S, Kołodziejczyk I, Gajda T et al. Manganese-induced Parkinsonism among ephedrone users and drug policy in Poland. *J Addict Med* 2013;7:302–3.

Grosset DG, Macphee GJ, Nairn M, on behalf of the Guideline Development Group. Diagnosis and pharmacological management of Parkinson's disease: summary of SIGN guidelines. *BMJ* 2010;340:5614.

Grosset D, Taurah L, Burn DJ et al. A multicentre longitudinal observational study of changes in self-reported health status in people with Parkinson's disease left untreated at diagnosis. *J Neurol Neurosurg Psychiatry* 2007;78:465–9.

Hauser RA, Hsu A, Espay AJ et al. Extended-release carbidopa-levodopa (IPX)66 compared with immediate-release carbidopa-levodopa in patients with Parkinson's disease and motor fluctuations: a phase 3 randomised, double-blind trial. *Lancet Neurol* 2013;346–56.

Hauser RA, Rascol O, Olanow W, Stocchi F. Effects of long-term rasagiline treatment on time to key PD milestones: results from the ADAGIO follow-up (AFU) study [abstract]. *Mov Disord* 2014;29(Suppl 1):655

Horstink M, Tolosa E, Bonuccelli G et al. Review of the therapeutic management of Parkinson's disease. Report of a joint task force of the EFNS and the MDS-ES. Part I: early (uncomplicated) Parkinson's disease – Guideline 51. *Eur J Neurol* 2006;13:1170–85.

Horstink M, Tolosa E, Bonuccelli G et al. Review of the therapeutic management of Parkinson's disease. Report of a joint task force of the EFNS and the MDS-ES. Part II: late (complicated) Parkinson's disease – Guideline 52. *Eur J Neurol* 2006; 13:1186–202.

LeWitt P. Rotigotine: a viewpoint by Peter LeWitt. *CNS Drugs* 2005;19:983–4.

Martinez-Martin P, Reddy P, Katzenschlager R et al. EuroInf: a multicenter comparative observational study of apomorphine and levodopa infusion in Parkinson's disease. *Mov Disord* 2015;30:510–16.

Naidu Y, Chaudhuri KR. Transdermal rotigotine: a new non-ergot dopamine agonist for the treatment of Parkinson's disease. *Expert Opin Drug Deliv* 2007;4:111–18.

NICE. *Parkinson's disease in over 20s: diagnosis and management. Clinical guideline 35.* London: National Institute for Health and Care Excellence, June 2006. www.nice.org.uk/guidance/cg35, last accessed 03 May 2016.

Nutt JG. Continuous dopaminergic stimulation: is it the answer to the motor complications of levodopa? *Mov Disord* 2007;22:1–9.

Nyholm D, Askmark H, Gomes-Trolin C et al. Optimising levodopa pharmacokinetics: intestinal infusion versus oral sustained-release tablets. *Clin Neuropharmacol* 2003;26: 156–63.

Olanow W, Schapira AH, Rascol O. Continuous dopamine-receptor stimulation in early Parkinson's disease. *Trends Neurosci* 2000;23:S117–26.

Olanow CW, Watts RL, Koller WC. An algorithm (decision tree) for the management of Parkinson's disease (2001): treatment guidelines. *Neurology* 2001;56(11suppl5):S1–88.

Pahwa R, Lyons KE, Hauser RA et al. Randomized trial of IPX066, carbidopa/levodopa extended release, in early Parkinson's disease. *Parkinsonism Relat Disord* 2014;20:142–8.

Parkinson Study Group. A controlled trial of rasagiline in early Parkinson disease: the TEMPO study. *Arch Neurol* 2002;59:1937–43.

Parkinson Study Group. Dopamine transporter brain imaging to assess the effects of pramipexole vs levodopa on Parkinson disease progression. *JAMA* 2002;287:1653–61.

PD Med Collaborative Group. Long-term effectiveness of dopamine agonists and monoamine oxidase B inhibitors compared with levodopa as initial treatment for Parkinson's disease (PD MED): a large, open-label, pragmatic randomised trial. *Lancet* 2014;384:1196–205.

Pondal M, Marras C, Miyasaki J et al. Clinical features of dopamine agonist withdrawal syndrome in a movement disorders clinic. *J Neurol Neurosurg Psychiatry* 2013;84:130–5.

Rabinak CA, Nirenberg MJ. Dopamine agonist withdrawal syndrome in Parkinson disease. *Arch Neurol* 2010;67:58e63.

Rascol O, Brooks DJ, Korczyn AD et al. A five-year study of the incidence of dyskinesia in patients with early Parkinson's disease who were treated with ropinirole or levodopa. 056 Study Group. *N Engl J Med* 2000;342:1484–91.

Rascol O, Goetz C, Koller W et al. Treatment interventions for Parkinson's disease: an evidence based assessment. *Lancet* 2002;359:1589–98.

Rusz J, Megrelishvili M, Bonnet C et al. A distinct variant of mixed dysarthria reflects parkinsonism and dystonia due to ephedrone abuse. *J Neural Transm* 2014;121:655–64.

Scottish Intercollegiate Guidelines Network (SIGN). *Diagnosis and Pharmacological Management of Parkinson's Disease: A National Clinical Guideline* (113). Edinburgh: Scottish Intercollegiate Guidelines Network, 2010.

Seppi K, Weintraub D, Coelho M et al. The Movement Disorder Society evidence-based medicine review update: treatments for the non-motor symptoms of Parkinson's disease. *Mov Disord* 2011;26:S42–80.

Stacy M, Bowron A, Guttman M et al. Identification of motor and nonmotor wearing off in Parkinson's disease: comparison of a patient questionnaire versus a clinician assessment. *Mov Disord* 2005;20:726–33.

Stocchi F, Vacca L, Ruggieri S, Olanow CW. Intermittent vs continuous levodopa administration in patients with advanced Parkinson's disease: a clinical and pharmacokinetic study. *Arch Neurol* 2005;62:905–10.

Swinn LA, James CR, Quinn NP, Lees AJ. *Treatment of Parkinson's Disease with Apomorphine. Shared Care Guidelines*, 5th edn. London: University College London Hospitals NHS Foundation Trust, 2005.

Trenkwalder C, Chaudhuri KR, Martinez-Martin P et al. Prolonged-release oxycodone–naloxone for treatment of severe pain in patients with Parkinson's disease (PANDA): a double-blind, randomised, placebo-controlled trial. *Lancet Neurol* 2015;14:1161–70.

Trenkwalder C, Kies B, Rudzinska M et al. and the RECOVER study group. Rotigotine effects on early morning motor function and sleep in Parkinson's disease: a double-blind, randomized, placebo-controlled study (RECOVER). *Mov Disord* 2011;26:90–9.

Van der Marck MA, Munneke M, Mulleners W et al; IMPACT study group. Integrated multidisciplinary care in Parkinson's disease: a non-randomised, controlled trial (IMPACT). *Lancet Neurol* 2013;12:947–56.

Weiss H, Marsh L. Impulse control disorders and compulsive behaviors associated with dopaminergic therapies in Parkinson disease *Neurol Clin Pract* 2012;2:267–74.

Zesiewicz TA, Sullivan KL, Arnulf I, et al. Practice parameter: treatment of nonmotor symptoms of Parkinson disease. Report of the Quality Standards Subcommittee of the American Academy of Neurology. *Neurology* 2010;74:924–31.

History

During the 1930s, neurosurgeons attempted to relieve Parkinson's disease symptoms by open brain surgery. The observation that hemiplegic stroke relieved Parkinson's disease tremor on the hemiplegic side led to surgery on the motor tract (Table 5.1). Although these operations were successful at controlling tremor, inevitably they led to paralysis of the affected side and were therefore abandoned.

Irving Cooper's remarkable serendipity is worth recounting: he was attempting pedunculotomy for parkinsonism, when bleeding occurred. The operation was abandoned but the patient improved substantially. Cooper had clipped the anterior choroidal artery, the main blood

TABLE 5.1

History of surgery for Parkinson's disease (excluding pedunculopontine stimulation)

Operation	Reference
Pyramidal tract	
Pyramidal tractotomy of cervical cord	Putnam 1940
Cerebral cortex excision	Bucy and Buchanan 1932; Klemme 1940
Cerebral peduncle incision	Walker 1952
Basal ganglia	
Caudate nucleus, globus pallidus lesions	Meyers 1942
Anterior choroidal artery ligation, chemopallidectomy, chemothalamotomy	Cooper 1954
Thalamotomy (ventral-intermediate nucleus)	Narabayashi and Ohye 1978
Pallidotomy	Laitinen et al. 1992
Subthalamotomy (dorsolateral)	Gill et al. 1997

supply to the globus pallidus. Following this, he embarked on a series of operations creating lesions within the globus pallidus and thalamus.

Physiological recording in the thalamus established the ventral-intermediate (VIM) nucleus as the source of tremor. Stereotactic thalamotomy became the most frequently performed operation for Parkinson's disease during the early 1960s because of its profound effect on tremor. However, by the mid-1960s, neurosurgery for Parkinson's disease had almost disappeared because of the introduction of levodopa. When the long-term problems with drug therapy, such as dyskinesias and drug-induced 'on/off' fluctuations, became apparent, the merits of neurosurgery were re-evaluated. This was influenced in particular by Laitinen in 1992, when he reported that his results using pallidotomy (surgery on the globus pallidus) over 20 years indicated sustained benefit.

In addition to lesional 'destruction' surgery, neuronal transplantation was attempted during the 1980s and experimental programs continue. More recently, deep brain stimulation using depth electrodes has been introduced.

Which patients require surgery?

Surgery is usually employed in patients when manipulations of drug therapy have failed to control 'off' symptoms, tremor, motor fluctuations and dyskinesias. It has a morbidity of approximately 2% from strokes and infection, and a mortality of about 0.5%, and may be an unpleasant experience. However, in carefully selected patients surgery leads to control of 'off' symptoms, motor fluctuations and dyskinesias.

Patients, their relatives and carers need to understand the limit of any benefits from an operation, and that surgery is not a cure. Sometimes patients are inclined to concentrate on an 'apparent' cure, such as surgery, when actually psychosocial concerns and dysfunctional family relationships are the main issues affecting their quality of life. Surgery will benefit a select number of patients, mostly those with young-onset Parkinson's disease who have had the disease for many years and who have 'on/off' syndromes. For these patients, the operation of choice is deep brain stimulation of the subthalamus to enable a reduction in dopaminergic therapy and control of dyskinesias.

Patients with severe resistant unilateral tremor may undergo single-side thalamic stimulation. Bilateral pallidal stimulation may be a treatment option for those with severe resistant dyskinesias but with limitations concerning age and neuropsychiatric risk profile for subthalamic stimulation. In some countries, subthalamic lesional surgery has been employed but it requires long-term evaluation before it can be recommended.

Today, most movement-disorder centers have an allied surgical program. It is not yet possible to say with certainty which patients benefit most from surgery and which operations should be performed. Ideally, surgical centers should take part in collaborative trials to evaluate the potential of lesional surgery and compare this older technique with deep brain stimulation.

Lesional surgery

Lesional surgery may be preferred to deep brain stimulation when a simpler procedure without complex follow-up is required, especially when it is suspected that a patient will not attend the necessary follow-up after insertion of a stimulator, or if patients have to travel long distances. In some parts of the world, the prohibitive cost of the stimulator (about US$32 000/£20 000 for hardware and follow-up) may lead to a preference for lesional surgery.

Lesional surgery is performed by stereotaxy (Figure 5.1). MRI and other neuroimaging methods are insufficient to place a lesion accurately and should be combined with physiological assessment. The patient is therefore woken at the time of lesional placement for physiological stimulation and microelectrode recording. Usually the lesion is created by thermocoagulation; however, cryosurgery is an alternative.

Pallidotomy, a procedure that involves destruction of part of the globus pallidus, is appropriate when there is severe dyskinesia (Table 5.2). Dyskinesias contralateral to the lesion may be greatly alleviated. Pharmacological adjustments are made postoperatively so that 'on' time can be increased. There is a 70% reduction in contralateral tremor and a 30% reduction in activities of daily living score, which allows some patients to return to functional independence.

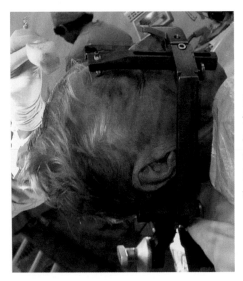

Figure 5.1 Stereotactic frame in place. The frame acts as an external three-dimensional reference for localization of structures within the brain.

TABLE 5.2

Pallidotomy (rarely performed)

Indications
- Severe unilateral dyskinesia

Contraindications
- Cognitive decline
- Neuropsychiatric problems, e.g. persistent hallucinations, depression
- Previous brain surgery
- Medical problems, e.g. cerebrovascular disease

Bilateral pallidotomy should be avoided because there is a high risk (≤ 10%) of speech and memory disorders. If a second operation is needed on the other side, it should be performed at a later time, and deep brain stimulation should be used in order to avoid permanent side effects. Given the evidence base for the safety and efficacy of subthalamic nucleus (STN) stimulation in patients with Parkinson's disease (see pages 103–8), pallidotomy is rarely performed nowadays.

Thalamotomy, surgery on the VIM nucleus of the thalamus, is the most effective way of controlling tremor. It can be used when tremor is the major disabling feature of Parkinson's disease, and also for essential or ataxic (Holmes') tremor. Deep brain stimulation is the best method of delivery, particularly if a bilateral operation is required. The complication rate is the same as for pallidotomy. Thalamotomy can effectively relieve tremor in 90% of cases, but it should be remembered that tremor is not usually a disabling feature of Parkinson's disease, and thalamotomy has no effect on bradykinesia.

Subthalamotomy is surgery on the STN, the main outflow tract of the basal ganglia, which is abnormally active in Parkinson's disease. Lesional surgery of the STN can improve tremor, bradykinesia and rigidity. Its effect can be compared with continuous apomorphine infusion, but it causes less dyskinesia. Care needs to be taken not to provoke dyskinesias or hemiballism. Subthalamotomy may carry a greater complication rate than other lesional surgery performed at the basal ganglia and is not generally recommended.

Deep brain stimulation

The hypothesis that deep brain stimulation (Table 5.3) could inhibit tremor and dyskinesias was proposed when it was found that electrical impulses applied during preoperative testing had this effect. The technology was already available from pain pathway stimulation. Alim Benabid's group in France has pioneered this approach in different movement disorders since 1987. Deep brain stimulation can be used to create electrical depolarization of neurons in any basal ganglia site.

The procedure. Electrodes are placed in basal ganglia targets using stereotaxy. Initially, wires emerging from the skull are attached to an external stimulator (Figure 5.2). The optimal level of stimulation is achieved when symptoms contralateral to placement are controlled with minimal side effects (such as visual field fluctuation or paresthesias). An internal stimulator is inserted subcutaneously below the clavicle and connected to a wire tunnelled subcutaneously from the scalp (Figure 5.3). Non-rechargeable batteries can last up to 5 years

TABLE 5.3

Deep brain stimulation

Indications	Contraindications

• Subthalamic stimulation
  – resistant motor fluctuations
  – drug-resistant dyskinesias
  – ? early motor complications (EARLYSTIM study)
• Thalamic stimulation
  – tremor: parkinsonian, essential/familial, ataxic (Holmes')
• Pallidal stimulation
  – as for subthalamic stimulation
	• Cognitive decline/ neuropsychiatric problems
	• Severe medical problems
	• Patient/carer non-adherence
	• Atypical parkinsonism
	• Gait freezing and postural instability while 'on'
	• Uncontrolled depression

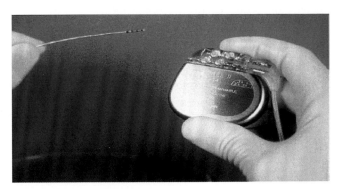

Figure 5.2 Stimulator box and wire.

and may be conserved by turning stimulation off at night; the patient can do this using a magnet. Rechargeable batteries can last for up to 25 years. Patients undergoing deep brain stimulation need to be followed up by a team able to monitor and adjust its effects.

Outcomes. Thalamic targets (VIM nucleus) are used for tremor, whether parkinsonian, essential or ataxic (Holmes'), and can provide

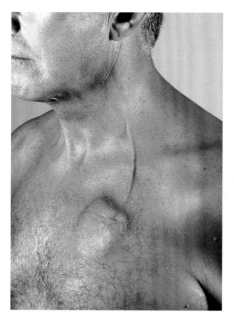

Figure 5.3 Stimulator in place with visible subcutaneous wire.

spectacular results. Tremor will cease within seconds of starting stimulation and reappears quickly on stopping. VIM deep brain stimulation appears not to be affected by age. The frequency of distal appendicular tremor and greater tremor indicates good control of tremor by VIM deep brain stimulation. Nevertheless, the STN is now the preferred target for control of parkinsonian signs. Deep brain stimulation can reverse akinesia, rigidity and tremor but not many axial symptoms. Stimulation of the globus pallidus does not control tremor but has a good effect on akinesia, rigidity and dyskinesia, with a smaller risk of neuropsychiatric side effects than STN stimulation.

A meta-analysis of outcomes from cohorts of patients undergoing deep brain stimulation of the STN suggests that dyskinesia is reduced by 69.1% (95% CI: 62–76.2%), the daily 'off' period is reduced by 68.2% (95% CI: 58–79%) and health-related quality of life is improved by $34.5 \pm 15.3\%$. Most studies have excluded patients over the age of 75 years.

Adverse events. The most common serious adverse event is intracranial hemorrhage (in 3.9% of patients), and psychiatric sequelae are common. Infection rates have an incidence of 1.6%, and replacement of portions of the device is needed in 4.4% of patients.

The VA trial comparing stimulation of the STN with that of the globus pallidus in patients with Parkinson's disease showed that the motor improvement was similar in the two targets but certain cognitive functions and depression worsened after STN stimulation. The researchers concluded that non-motor symptoms should be considered when choosing the target for deep brain stimulation in Parkinson's disease; up to now, deep brain stimulation has primarily focused on motor symptoms. Non-motor symptoms are common, present in early and advanced stages of the disease and have a huge effect on patients' health-related quality of life. They therefore need to be addressed by every treatment offered to patients with Parkinson's disease.

Effect on non-motor symptoms. Long-term follow up of carefully selected patients indicates that STN deep brain stimulation is a safe procedure with regard to most non-motor symptoms. The number and severity of some non-motor symptoms decrease significantly after STN deep brain stimulation, resulting in a significant improvement in quality of life and activities of daily living.

However, not all non-motor symptoms improve; indeed, some may deteriorate both transiently and permanently. Worsening of non-motor symptoms, especially in the neuropsychological and psychiatric domains, is most often seen transiently in the immediate postoperative period after STN deep brain stimulation, possibly related to the changes in dopamine replacement therapy or the surgery itself.

Quality of life and mortality. A large randomized study by Deuschl et al. demonstrated that subthalamic neurostimulation resulted in a significant and clinically meaningful improvement in the quality of life of patients under 75 years of age with advanced Parkinson's disease who had severe fluctuations in mobility and dyskinesia. The patients who received neurostimulation had longer periods with less dyskinesia and better-quality mobility. In the EARLYSTIM study (see below), STN deep brain stimulation had the same positive effects on motor function, fluctuations and quality of life in patients with a much earlier stage of Parkinson's disease.

The changes in motor function in patients with advanced Parkinson's disease also led to improvement in activities of daily living and quality of life (emotional wellbeing, stigma and bodily discomfort). Cognition, mood and overall psychiatric functioning were unchanged. The authors concluded that, in carefully selected patients, neurostimulation of the STN is a powerful treatment that alleviates the burden of Parkinson's disease. The prospect of an improved quality of life in patients treated with neurostimulation has to be weighed against the risk of complications related to surgery.

A further study by Schupbach and colleagues examined the effect of deep brain stimulation on mortality in Parkinson's disease, by examining the records of 171 consecutive cases treated by deep brain stimulation of the STN. Poor preoperative cognitive function appeared to be a predictive factor for mortality, while survival among patients who underwent surgery was no better than those who did not have the operation.

EARLYSTIM. In the 2-year EARLYSTIM study, 251 patients with Parkinson's disease and early motor complications (mean age 52 years; mean duration of disease 7.5 years) were randomly assigned to STN stimulation plus medical therapy or medical therapy alone. The primary endpoint of the study was quality of life measured by the Parkinson's Disease Questionnaire (PDQ-39) summary index (higher scores indicating worse function).

Quality of life scores improved by 7.8 points in the surgical group and worsened by 0.2 points in the medical group (mean between-group difference from baseline to 2 years, 8.0 points; $p = 0.002$). Neurostimulation was found to be superior to medical therapy with respect to motor disability ($p < 0.001$), activities of daily living ($p < 0.001$) and levodopa-induced motor complications ($p < 0.001$).

Adverse events. Serious adverse events were reported in 54.8% of the surgical arm and 44.1% of the medical arm. The authors concluded that STN stimulation was superior to conventional medical treatment in patients with Parkinson's disease with early motor complications. However, there is still controversy regarding the study group's patient selection and whether patients in the medical arm were given the best medical therapy available such as apomorphine or intrajejunal levodopa infusion.

Nerve-cell transplantation
Attempts to transplant nervous tissue in animals have been made since the 1890s (Table 5.4). Successful transplantation of fetal mesencephalic dopamine neurons was achieved in 1987 (Figure 5.4). Over 500 patients worldwide have now received nerve-cell transplants into the brain.

Aborted 6–10-week-old fetuses are harvested and dissected for midbrain dopamine cells. These are either dispersed in enzymatic solution or injected as clumps of cells. Cells from up to four fetuses are needed for stereotactic injection into eight sites in both hemispheres (caudate and putaminal nuclei).

TABLE 5.4

History of nerve-cell transplantation

Operation	Reference
Unsuccessful transplantation of cortex between cats and dogs	Thompson 1890
Successful transplantation of fetal rat tissue	Dunn 1917
Graft survival of rat nervous tissue	May 1955
Reversal of behavioral changes in rat parkinsonian model	Björklund and Stenevi 1979
Unsuccessful transplantation of adrenal medulla in a human patient with Parkinson's disease	Backlund et al. 1985
Reversal of monkey parkinsonism	Redmond et al. 1986
Implantation of fetal mesencephalon in a human patient with Parkinson's disease	Henderson et al. 1991
Negative results for sham-controlled studies of human fetal transplantation	Freed et al. 2001, Olanow et al. 2003
Neuronal allotransplantation with fetal ventral mesencephalic tissue (TRANSEURO)	Open-label study under way

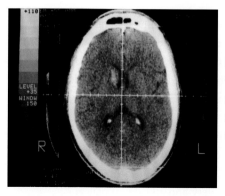

Figure 5.4 CT scan following transplantation of fetal mesencephalic tissue into the right caudate head of a patient with Parkinson's disease.

Patients are given immunosuppressive therapy with ciclosporin and prednisolone (prednisone) for up to 6 months, although whether this is necessary has not been established. The aim is to restore lost dopamine cells. So far, results indicate that implanted cells can survive, grow and form dendritic connections with host neurons.

Autopsy has revealed dopaminergic differentiation of these cells and clinically there have been individual successes, with reversal of motor signs and cessation of dopa drugs. However, in the first controlled trial by Freed et al. in 2001, involving 40 patients randomized to fetal neural transplant or sham surgery, primary outcome measures failed to show any significant differences between the two groups. Furthermore, about 15% of the transplant patients developed severe facial dystonia and disabling 'runaway' dyskinesias.

In a controlled double-blind study reported by Olanow et al. in 2003, 34 patients were randomized to either fetal neural transplant with two volumes of donor tissue or sham surgery. Primary outcome measures again failed to show any significant differences between the two groups, and 56% of transplant patients developed dyskinesias. The authors commented that fetal nigral transplantation cannot be recommended as treatment for Parkinson's disease.

There is hope that cell implantation may replace dopa therapy, but this has not yet been realized. Other sources of cells will need to be found if the technique is to become generalized. Immortalized neural stem-cell lines are in development, and porcine fetal cells are undergoing trials but may carry the additional risk of introducing porcine viruses into humans.

The problem remains that even successfully implanted cells may die in the same way as the replaced cells. Research into the rewiring of the human nervous system is ongoing, but it will be decades before a recognized treatment is available. In addition, there is evidence to suggest the possibility of a transmissible prion-like pathology.

TRANSEURO study. European researchers are trying to develop an efficacious and safe treatment methodology for Parkinson's disease using fetal cell-based therapies. The investigators have started an open-label study to assess the safety and efficacy of neural allotransplantation with fetal ventral mesencephalic tissue in patients with Parkinson's disease; the results are awaited.

Glial cell-line-derived neurotrophic factor
Glial cell-line-derived neurotrophic factor (GDNF) is a protein that stimulates cell signaling pathways that regulate dopaminergic neuronal survival, differentiation, growth and regeneration in vitro, and has been shown to have protective effects on dopaminergic neurons in animal models. Several studies have shown that infusion of GDNF into the brain of parkinsonian mice treated with 1-methyl-4-phenyl-1,2,3,6-tetrahydropyridine (MPTP) improved motor function. Postmortem examination of the mice brains showed partial restoration of dopamine in the corpus striatum and dopaminergic fibers in the substantia nigra. However, evidence for the safety and effectiveness of GDNF in humans is lacking.

In 1999, Kordower et al. reported 1 patient with a 23-year history of Parkinson's disease who developed side effects after intraventricular infusion of GDNF, with no improvement in parkinsonian symptoms and no evidence at postmortem examination of regeneration. An open-label phase 1 safety trial in 5 patients with Parkinson's disease showed an improvement in 'off' state and dyskinesias after 1 year, with a 28% increase in putaminal 18-fluorodopa uptake on positron emission tomography (PET) scans. However, a subsequent phase 2 double-blind placebo-controlled study in 34 patients with advanced Parkinson's disease failed to show any clinical benefit.

Currently, there is concern that GDNF infusion may cause cerebellar lesions, as seen in animal models. However, a placebo-controlled randomized double-blind trial is under way in the UK to assess the safety and efficacy of intermittent bilateral intraputaminal GDNF infusions administered via convection enhanced delivery (CED) in patients with Parkinson's disease.

Platelet-derived growth factor

Platelet-derived growth factor (PDGF), also known as sNN0031 (becaplermin), is a recombinant human platelet-derived growth factor BB (rhPDGF-BB) administered by short-term continuous infusion into the ventricular lumen using an implantable pump and brain catheter. Initial trials to assess the tolerability and efficacy of intracerebroventricular administration of sNN0031 in patients with idiopathic Parkinson's disease have been discontinued, but this treatment may have application in clinical trials in the future.

Retinal cell transplantation

Retinal pigment epithelium (RPE) is a source of dopamine, and transplantation into the basal ganglia could potentially form a new therapy for Parkinson's disease. In-vitro rat models using a conditioned medium derived from RPE resulted in increased neuritic growth of 78% in striatal neurons, suggesting a potential benefit of RPE transplantation in Parkinson's disease.

One small open-label study in 6 patients, involving unilateral stereotactic putaminal transplantation of RPE cells attached to biocompatible microcarriers, showed a 34% improvement in the primary outcome measure. A randomized trial involving 72 patients showed no statistically significant difference in the 'off' state between RPE- and sham-implanted patients at 12 months. There were also no differences in secondary outcomes, including 'on'-state Unified Parkinson's Disease Rating Scale (UPDRS) III, time spent in 'off' or 'on' state, levodopa reduction or UPDRS activities of daily living score.

Key points – neurosurgery

• Surgery is recommended when optimal drug treatment options have failed to control symptoms.

• Neurosurgery is an unpleasant experience for the patient; the main complications are stroke and infection.

• For patients with young-onset Parkinson's disease who have had 'on/off' symptoms for many years, the procedure of choice is deep brain stimulation of the subthalamic nucleus to reduce dopaminergic therapy and control dyskinesias.

• Lesional surgery is an alternative to deep brain stimulation for patients unlikely to attend regular follow-up or who have to travel long distances, or in instances where the cost of a stimulator is prohibitive.

• Pallidotomy is appropriate for severe dyskinesia.

• Thalamic deep brain surgery (VIM nucleus) is the most effective procedure for controlling parkinsonian tremor.

• In the future, nerve-cell transplantation could replace dopaminergic treatment if sources of dopamine cells other than 6–10-week-old fetuses can be found; trials using porcine fetal cells, stem cells that generate dopamine and other such cells (e.g. retinal cells) are under way.

Key references

Ashkan K, Wallace B, Bell BA et al. Deep brain stimulation of the subthalamic nucleus in Parkinson's disease 1993-2003: where are we 10 years on? *Br J Neurosurg* 2004;18:19–34.

Backlund EO, Granberg PO, Hamberger B et al. Transplantation of adrenal medullary tissue to striatum in parkinsonism. First clinical trials. *J Neurosurg* 1985;62:169–73.

Benabid AL, Deuschl G, Lang AE et al. Deep brain stimulation for Parkinson's disease. *Mov Disord* 2006;21(suppl14):S168–70.

Benabid AL, Pollak P, Louveau A et al. Combined (thalamotomy and stimulation) stereotactic surgery of the VIM thalamic nucleus for bilateral Parkinson's disease. *Appl Neurophysiol* 1987;50:344–6.

Björklund A, Stenevi U. Reconstruction of the nigrostriatal dopamine pathway by intracerebral nigral transplants. *Brain Res* 1979;177:555–60.

Brundin P. GDNF treatment in Parkinson's disease: time for controlled clinical trials? *Brain* 2002;125:2149–51.

Bucy PC, Buchanan DN. Athetosis. *Brain* 1932;55:479–92.

Burton EA, Glorioso JC, Fink DJ. Gene therapy progress and prospects: Parkinson's disease. *Gene Ther* 2003;10:1721–7.

Cooper IS. Surgical alleviation of Parkinsonism: effects of occlusion of the anterior choroidal artery. *J Am Geriatr Soc* 1954;2:691–718.

Cooper IS. 20-year followup study of the neurosurgical treatment of dystonia musculorum deformans. *Adv Neurol* 1976;14:423–52.

Cooper IS, Riklan M. Cryothalamectomy for abnormal movement disorders. *St Barnabas Hosp Med Bull* 1962;1:17–23.

Deuschl G, Schade-Brittinger C, Krack P et al. A randomized trial of deep-brain stimulation for Parkinson's disease. *N Engl J Med* 2006;355:896–908.

Dunn EH. Primary and secondary findings in a series of attempts to transplant cerebral cortex in the albino rat. *J Comp Neurol* 1917;27:565–82.

Fasano A, Daniele A, Albanese A. Treatment of motor and non-motor features of Parkinson's disease with deep brain stimulation. *Lancet Neurol* 2012;11:429–42.

Freed CR, Greene PE, Breeze RE et al. Transplantation of embryonic dopamine neurons for severe Parkinson's disease. *N Engl J Med* 2001;344:710–19.

Grondin R, Zhang Z, Yi A et al. Chronic, controlled GDNF infusion promotes structural and functional recovery in advanced parkinsonian monkeys. *Brain* 2002;125: 2191–201.

Henderson BT, Clough CG, Hughes RC et al. Implantation of human fetal ventral mesencephalon to the right caudate nucleus in advanced Parkinson's disease. *Arch Neurol* 1991;48:822–7.

Klemme RM. Surgical treatment of dystonia, paralysis agitans and athetosis. *Arch Neurol Psychiatry* 1940;44:926.

Klingelhoefer L, Samuel M, Chaudhuri KR et al. An update of the impact of deep brain stimulation on non motor symptoms in Parkinson's disease. *J Parkinsons Dis* 2014;4:289–300.

Kordower JH, Emborg ME, Bloch J et al. Neurodegeneration prevented by lentiviral vector delivery of GDNF in primate models of Parkinson's disease. *Science* 2000;290:767–73.

Kordower JH, Palfi S, Chen EY et al. Clinicopathological findings following intraventricular glial-derived neurotrophic factor treatment in a patient with Parkinson's disease. *Ann Neurol* 1999;46:419–24.

Laitinen LV, Bergenheim AT, Hariz MI. Leksell's posteroventral pallidotomy in the treatment of Parkinson's disease. *J Neurosurg* 1992;76:53–61.

Madrazo I, Leon V, Torres C et al. Transplantation of fetal substantia nigra and adrenal medulla to the caudate nucleus in two patients with Parkinson's disease. *N Engl J Med* 1988;318:51.

May RM. Cerebral transplantation in mammals. *Transplantation Bull* 1955;2:62.

Meyers R. The modification of alternating tremors, rigidity and festination by surgery of the basal ganglia. *Res Publ Ass Res Nerv Ment Dis* 1942;21:602–65.

Narabayashi H. Surgical approach to tremor. In: Marsden CD, Fahn S, eds. *Movement Disorders*. London: Butterworth Scientific, 1982:292–9.

Narabayashi H, Ohye C. Parkinsonian tremor and nucleus ventralis intermedius of the human thalamus. *Prog Clin Neurophysiol* 1978;5:165–72.

Olanow CW, Goetz CG, Kordower JH et al. A double-blind controlled trial of bilateral fetal nigral transplantation in Parkinson's disease. *Ann Neurol* 2003;54:403–14.

Putnam TJ. Treatment of unilateral paralysis agitans by section of the lateral pyramidal tract. *Arch Neurol Psychiatry* 1940;44:950–76.

Redmond DE, Sladek JR Jr, Roth RH et al. Fetal neuronal grafts in monkeys given methylphenyltetra-hydropyridine. *Lancet* 1986;1:1125–7.

Schupbach MW, Rau J, Knudsen K et al. Neurostimulation for Parkinson's disease with early motor complications. *N Engl J Med* 2013;368:610–22.

Schupbach MW, Welter ML, Bonnet AM et al. Mortality in patients with Parkinson's disease treated by stimulation of the subthalamic nucleus. *Mov Disord* 2007;22:257–61.

Stover NP, Bakay RA, Subramanian T et al. Intrastriatal implantation of human retinal pigment epithelial cells attached to microcarriers in advanced Parkinson's disease. *Arch Neurol* 2005;62:1833–7.

Thompson WG. Successful brain grafting. *N Y Med J* 1890;51:701–2.

Walker AE. Cerebral pedunculotomy for the relief of involuntary movements. II. Parkinsonian tremor. *J Nerv Ment Dis* 1952;116:766–75.

Wolz M, Hauschild J, Fauser M et al. Immediate effects of deep brain stimulation of the subthalamic nucleus on nonmotor symptoms in Parkinson's disease. *Parkinsonism Relat Disord* 2012;18:994-7.

A multidisciplinary approach is an absolute requirement for optimal care of the parkinsonian patient. Early on, the main requirement is for information and counseling. In the later stages of the disease, coordination of the various agencies involved in care is often difficult and, as time passes, additional agencies will have to be accessed by the treating physician (Table 6.1). Many patients find the support offered by organizations such as Parkinson's UK helpful (see Useful resources, pages 161–3). A Parkinson's disease nurse specialist (PDNS) can spend more time with the patient and can offer telephone support. Some patients may need specialist counseling to help them to come to terms with the diagnosis.

Parkinson's disease nurse specialist. The PDNS is a key and essential member of the Parkinson's disease care team; they are usually the first point of contact for the patient, both within the hospital and at home.

TABLE 6.1

Agencies and professionals involved in the care of the parkinsonian patient

- Carer support network
- Family practitioner, geriatrician or neurologist
- Parkinson's disease nurse specialist
- Community- or hospital-based therapist, e.g. physiotherapist, speech and language therapist, occupational therapist, dietitian, continence advisor
- Community (district) nurse
- Psychiatrist, psychologist, specialist counselor (e.g. sex therapist)
- Pharmacist
- Local hospital (acute admission)
- Nursing home, if home care is impossible

The PDNS is skilled in patient and carer assessment, differential diagnosis of Parkinson's disease and appropriate drug treatment, medicines management and communication. The role of the PDNS in the care of patients with Parkinson's disease has been reported in three randomized controlled trials (RCTs), although the methods used in these studies have varied widely. The studies reported that PDNS care allowed a swift implementation of good clinical practice for Parkinson's disease, including home visits, and a high rate of patient satisfaction.

Ongoing support

In the early stages, the main focus is often on drug therapy. This should be initiated following specialist advice, but the family physician or PDNS may provide continuing supervision provided there is good liaison with the specialist (neurologist or geriatrician). Therapists have a useful role at all stages of the disease and should work as part of the multidisciplinary team.

Physiotherapists can advise on exercise, stretches, postural corrections, gait supervision and strategies for dealing with falls. Walking aids are usually unhelpful, but when falls and fear of falling emerge walking sticks are often adopted. Wheeled delta frames with brakes are better than static frames and allow fluent walking movement when falls become a problem. Despite this, some patients will need a wheelchair outside the home. However, early use of a wheelchair may indicate an alternative diagnosis.

"The ongoing physiotherapy I receive is a great help in keeping me mobile and fighting the rigidity."

The role of physiotherapy in Parkinson's disease has been examined to a reasonable extent in randomized trials, although a robust evidence base is still lacking. In a Cochrane review of data from 11 randomized trials, four reported a significant improvement in 280 patients after physiotherapy directed at the limbs and trunk for 8–30 hours over 3–52 weeks.

Other studies have addressed small numbers of patients only; for example, one randomized trial evaluated 8 patients in a 16-week aerobic exercise program. In another, 88 patients were randomized to the Alexander technique, massage or a control group. Significant improvements were reported in outcome measures in treated patients versus controls at 6 months.

Home exercise programs are popular with patients with Parkinson's disease as they can be tailored to their individual needs and practiced within the safety and comfort of their own home. A recent study has reported that approximately 79% of prescribed exercises are adhered to.

Physiotherapy in Parkinson's disease is currently recommended to educate patients about gait, initiation of movement and balance, as well as providing advice on safety within the home environment. As such, these interventions are very useful as the condition advances and balance problems, along with fear of falling, become apparent.

Speech and language therapists can advise on speech exercises and can encourage communication if patients are ignored or feel left out of conversations. In the later stages of disease, speech and language therapists may need to advise on swallowing difficulties, as well as food composition and consistency. If choking is a problem, liquids may be thickened and food homogenized.

The evidence base of efficacy for speech and language therapy (SALT) is limited by the small numbers of patients included in trials: three RCTs have evaluated a total sample of 63 patients. One study investigated the use of Lee Silverman Voice Treatment (LSVT), a speech therapy program comprising 16 1-hour sessions, which was developed in North America with the aim of restoring oral communication in patients with Parkinson's disease.

The majority of positive outcomes reported after SALT involve the use of LSVT.

"I have no doubts that the LSVT program has been of great benefit in maintaining the volume and clarity of my speech."

117

Occupational therapists should be involved if there is difficulty with daily living activities. Adaptation of the home is often necessary when the patient becomes more disabled. For example, ramps and widened doorways will allow wheelchair access, and a shower rather than a bath will allow the patient to sit on a stool and wash.

Occupational therapists assess the safety of homes, particularly when the patient is prone to falling. Grab-rails can be fitted, sharp corners protected, and patients can wear hip protectors to prevent hip fractures. Social services may need to be involved to make such changes and to assess the need for financial assistance.

In the past, there has been little evidence to support the use of interventional occupational therapy for patients with Parkinson's disease; however, new studies have shown efficacy. A recent RCT reported a self-perceived increase in the performance of daily activities when participating in individualized occupational therapy in the home. There has also been a Cochrane review of the efficacy of occupational therapy in 84 people in two randomized parallel-group trials. One trial reported continued maintenance of the Barthel index score (a measure of activities of daily living) over a 1-year period in patients who received occupational therapy.

Carers. Often the brunt of care falls on a patient's spouse or partner. Additional help may be needed to assist the patient with dressing, toileting or bathing. Consultations with the patient should include the carer, with attention given to the carer's mental and physical health and to whether additional support is needed.

Patients who hallucinate or have dementia often provoke social crises and cries for help from carers. Hallucinations may be temporary and related to excessive drug treatment, but often presage cognitive decline with memory difficulties and disorientation. These are the most difficult problems for patients with Parkinson's disease and their carers, and occur in at least 30% of cases. Swift action is required, and the availability of a PDNS is often invaluable.

The first step is to rationalize drug treatment, removing those drugs that are least effective or most likely to cause hallucinosis.

Therapy with levodopa plus a decarboxylase inhibitor is often the best policy. Neuroleptics that may aggravate parkinsonism should be avoided.

Support from nurses and social services is vital in keeping patients at home as long as possible, because admission to hospital in this situation may further aggravate decline. Despite this, patients with dementia frequently cannot be managed at home and will need to be admitted to a nursing home, either for respite care or on a permanent basis. The PDNS can advise nursing homes on effective management of patients with Parkinson's disease who have dementia, and the importance of regulating their medication. Demented patients who are prone to wander may need a locked facility.

Diet

A healthy diet is recommended, with attention to overall nutrition and roughage. In the early stages of the disease, eating plenty of fruit and vegetables should be encouraged to stimulate a sluggish bowel. Advice from a dietitian may be needed if a patient's nutritional intake is thought to be poor. An early warning sign is when the patient does not finish meals. It may be necessary to liquidize food and to provide dietary supplements, although these are a last resort.

Constipation can be distressing and high-residue diets may make matters worse. Lactulose or another osmotic laxative is first-line treatment. They will make stools softer but may lead to incontinence. Bowel stimulation using senna can be useful, but more powerful drugs, and eventually suppositories and micro-enemas, may be needed. A double-blind placebo-controlled trial reported good efficacy for Movicol in the treatment of constipation in patients with Parkinson's disease.

Interaction of food with drugs. Patients often ask how food interferes with drug treatment. In theory, a large protein intake competes with levodopa absorption and thereby prevents the drug's action, but significant dietary changes are not usually required. Even without drug treatment patients often feel worse in the afternoon, which may be due, in part, to a fall in blood pressure after a large meal at lunchtime. 119

"Carers can make eating more pleasant for the patient by ensuring the meal is relatively easy to eat, and that no large pieces of meat are being served to avoid swallowing problems. Give the patient sufficient time to eat the meal, and keep the patient company at the table."

If there appears to be a clear-cut relationship between eating large meals and patient deterioration, then changes such as moving the main meal to the evening or eating more frequent smaller meals may help.

Patients should not restrict their total protein intake unless they demonstrate an unusual sensitivity to protein (e.g. interference with the levodopa response after a large protein meal). The overall aim should be to achieve a well-balanced diet.

Bladder symptoms

Bladder dysfunction has a significant effect on quality of life, so with 50% of patients showing significant bladder symptoms it is important that they are treated and managed appropriately. In men, symptoms mimic prostatism, although without flow disturbance or postmicturition dribble. In elderly men, symptoms are often a result of both Parkinson's disease and prostatic hypertrophy.

Transurethral resection of the prostate may lead to incontinence, so urodynamic studies and a careful assessment by the urologist are required before this operation is considered.

Treatment with anticholinergics, such as oxybutynin, 2.5 mg twice daily, can relieve urgency and frequency. However, the symptoms may be resistant in later disease and these drugs can cause side effects such as confusion, dry mouth and aggravation of prostatic outflow problems.

It is necessary to rule out additional urinary infection before any treatment. Antidiuretic hormone taken before going to bed at night may relieve nocturnal incontinence or frequency.

A continence nurse will be able to give invaluable advice and will provide continence pads and other appropriate items. Simple practical measures such as having a urinal or bedpan by the bed can also be helpful.

Skin care

Although skin problems related to parkinsonism are common, patients rarely complain about them. Seborrheic dermatitis may cause crusting of the scalp and can be treated with antifungal preparations. Skin lesions may be treated with combination creams that contain antifungals and hydrocortisone. Episodic sweating can be troublesome and is not easily treated, though anticholinergics such as benzhexol may be tried. Drug rashes are not uncommon, particularly with the use of dopamine agonists, and may necessitate withdrawal of the offending drug.

Sexual problems

Sexual problems are not uncommon and are usually the concern of male patients; these issues need to be addressed with the patient as they are often important in terms of overall quality of life. Early-onset erectile dysfunction may indicate an alternative diagnosis, such as multiple system atrophy (MSA), but also occurs in parkinsonism. Sexual problems can also result from relationship dysfunction (e.g. caused by fear of illness), apathy as part of cognitive decline or inappropriate sexual arousal as a result of drug treatment (particularly dopamine agonists and apomorphine).

Alternatively, neuropsychiatric problems as a result of cognitive decline and drug treatment can lead to delusional beliefs regarding spousal infidelity, which may not respond to changes in drug treatment, cognitive therapy or atypical neuroleptics.

Erectile dysfunction, if proven to be the cause of sexual difficulties (i.e. if early-morning erections fail), can be treated with sildenafil in the usual way, assuming there is no medical contraindication or significant hypotension, and provided there has been full discussion with the patient's partner.

Palliative (not terminal) care

The need for palliative care in Parkinson's disease indicates a stage when drugs are no longer well tolerated, the patient is an unsuitable candidate for surgery and there is considerable comorbidity. The burden of both motor and non-motor symptoms is high in the advanced stages of Parkinson's disease, such that patients may require specialist palliative care services to improve quality of life.

Palliative care addresses physical problems such as pain, breathlessness, loss of appetite, immobility and constipation, as well as the personal, psychosocial and spiritual needs of the patient and their family. Usually, the Parkinson's disease nurse or specialist will recognize this stage of the disease process and support and initiate the appropriate care with specialist palliative care professionals. At this stage, non-invasive non-oral dopaminergic therapies become very important. Many patients may benefit from cautious and monitored administration of the rotigotine transdermal patch or apomorphine infusion to help with immobility-related pain, stiffness and other problems such as risk of aspiration.

A randomized fast-track trial to evaluate the clinical- and cost-effectiveness of short-term integrated palliative care services for people with advanced long-term neurological conditions, including Parkinson's disease, is running in the UK. It aims to develop a palliative care outcome scale (IPOS Neuro-S8) that is specific to Parkinson's disease. 'End of Life' initiatives such as the one set up by the UK Department of Health train health professionals in the palliative needs and care of patients. However, it should be stressed that while early palliative intervention can be highly beneficial to patients' quality of life, the need for palliative care in Parkinson's disease does not mean an imminent end of life.

Planning ahead. For those people who are approaching the end of life (likely to die within the next 12 months), a holistic assessment that considers their changing needs and preferences should be offered, with the opportunity to discuss the results of disease progression and possible outcomes, and develop and review a personalized care plan for current and future support and treatment.

Complex decisions should be made when there is enough time for clear evaluation. Advance directives are legal documents that inform health professionals of the patient's wishes in various situations; for example, with respect to parenteral feeding, catheterization, treatment of infection and resuscitation. As individuals may reach a point where they are no longer deemed to have the capacity to make decisions about their own care, these decisions clearly need to be made in advance. Alternatively, power of attorney enables a spouse, parent or sibling to make decisions regarding care once the patient is no longer able to.

Respite for carers. The advanced stages of Parkinson's disease can be a particularly difficult time for carers, and it is important they are made aware of the support and respite care available to them (see Useful resources, pages 161–3).

Key points – other therapies and support

- Early in the course of the disease, patients most need clear information, advice and counseling.
- Multidisciplinary therapy and input from a Parkinson's disease nurse specialist (PDNS) should be available to all patients at all stages of the disease. The PDNS is ideally placed to recognize when palliative care is needed, and to initiate and support the appropriate care.
- Physiotherapy is particularly useful at a stage when balance problems become obvious.
- In early Parkinson's disease, patients should be encouraged to eat plenty of fruit and vegetables to stimulate a sluggish bowel.
- Although a large protein intake may compete with levodopa absorption, patients should not restrict their total protein intake.
- Hallucinations often presage cognitive decline with memory difficulties and disorientation, the most difficult problems for both patients and carers; drugs that are most likely to cause hallucinosis should be withdrawn immediately.
- Bladder symptoms, sleep problems and sexual problems are common, and need to be addressed.
- Skin problems are common, but patients rarely complain of them; drug rashes may necessitate withdrawal of the offending agent.
- Patients and carers should be given the chance to discuss end-of-life issues at the appropriate time with suitably trained professionals.

Key references

Baja NPS, Clough CG. Non-motor aspects of idiopathic Parkinson's disease. *Curr Med Lit Parkinson's Disease* 2001;3:1–6.

Chaudhuri KR, Healy D, Schapira AH. Non-motor symptoms of Parkinson's disease: diagnosis and management. *Lancet Neurol* 2006;5:235–45.

Deane KHO, Ellis-Hill C, Playford ED et al. Occupational therapy for Parkinson's disease. *Cochrane Database Syst Rev* 2001, issue 2. CD002813.

Deane KHO, Jones D, Ellis-Hill C et al. Physiotherapy for patients with Parkinson's disease: a comparison of techniques. *Cochrane Database Syst Rev* 2001, issue 1. CD002815.

Deane KHO, Whurr R, Playford ED et al. Speech and language therapy versus placebo or no intervention for dysarthria in Parkinson's disease. *Cochrane Database Syst Rev* 2001, issue 2. CD002812.

Deane KHO, Whurr R, Playford ED et al. Speech and language therapy for dysarthria in Parkinson's disease: a comparison of techniques. *Cochrane Database Syst Rev* 2001, issue 2. CD002814.

Eichhorn TE, Oertel WH. Macrogol 3350/electrolyte improves constipation in Parkinson's disease and multiple system atrophy. *Mov Disord* 2001;16:1176–7.

Jarman B, Hurwitz B, Cook A et al. Effects of community based nurses specialising in Parkinson's disease on health outcome and costs: randomised controlled trial. *BMJ* 2002;324:1072–5.

MacMahon DG, Thomas S. Practical approach to quality of life in Parkinson's disease: the nurse's role. *J Neurol* 1998;245(suppl 1):S19–22.

Pickering RM, Fritton C, Ballinger C et al. Self reported adherence to a home-based exercise programme among people with Parkinson's Disease. *Parkinsonism Rel Disord* 2013;19:66–71.

Quinn NP, Koller WC, Lang AE, Marsden CD. Painful Parkinson's disease. *Lancet* 1986;1:1366–9.

Saleem TZ, Higginson IJ, Chaudhuri KR et al. Symptom prevalence, severity and palliative care needs assessment using the Palliative Outcome Scale: a cross-sectional study of patients with Parkinson's disease and related neurological conditions. *Palliat Med* 2013;27:722–31.

Stallibrass C, Sissons P, Chalmers C. Randomized controlled trial of the Alexander technique for idiopathic Parkinson's disease. *Clin Rehabil* 2002;16:695–708.

Sturkenboom H, Graff MJ, Hendricks JC et al. Efficacy of occupational therapy for patients with Parkinson's disease: a randomised controlled trial. *Lancet Neurol* 2014;13:557–66.

Long-term complications develop in virtually all patients taking continued levodopa therapy. Although levodopa is the most effective drug for the treatment of Parkinson's disease, the initial benefit begins to diminish over time with dyskinesias and fluctuations in motor response (Figure 7.1). It is likely that two factors determine the development of fluctuations and dyskinesias:
• disease severity
• chronic pulsatile stimulation of postsynaptic dopamine receptors by the use of dopaminergic drugs with a short half-life.

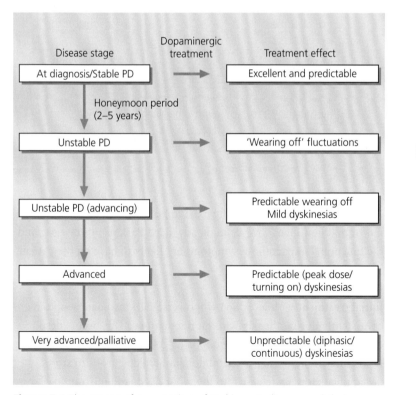

Figure 7.1 The stages of progression of Parkinson's disease and their relationship to motor complications.

TABLE 7.1

Ranking of the clinically most important indicators for patients suspected of having advanced Parkinson's disease

Rank	Motor symptoms	Non-motor symptoms	Functional impacts
1	Moderate level of troublesome fluctuations	Mild level of dementia	Repeated falls despite optimal treatment
2	At least 2 hours of the waking day with 'off' symptoms	Non-transitory troublesome hallucinations	Needs help with activities of daily living at least some of the time
3	At least 1 hour of the day with troublesome dyskinesias	Moderate level of psychosis	Not able to perform complex tasks at least some of the time
4	Moderate level of dyskinesias	Fluctuations	Moderately impaired mobility
5	Troublesome dysphagia	Moderate level of night-time sleep disturbances	
6	Daily oral levodopa doses '5 times a day'		

Table 7.1 shows the clinically most important indicators, both motor and non-motor, for defining advanced Parkinson's disease, and the functional impact those symptoms are likely to have on the patient.

Motor fluctuations

Initial treatment with levodopa will reverse parkinsonian symptoms consistently during the day without fluctuations. This occurs despite the short plasma half-life of levodopa (2–3 hours), and presumably reflects the ability of nigrostriatal dopaminergic neurons to store dopamine before its release into the synapse. Coadministration of a decarboxylase inhibitor, such as carbidopa or benserazide, prevents metabolism of levodopa to dopamine in the bloodstream. These drugs do not cross the blood–brain barrier, and so dopa is decarboxylated to dopamine within the neurons without rate limitation.

Established/unstable Parkinson's disease. Within 2–3 years, most patients begin to experience fluctuations (Table 7.2). In advanced disease, the improvement in parkinsonism correlates with the level of levodopa in the bloodstream (Table 7.3). One factor underlying the development of fluctuations is the progressive fallout of dopamine neurons within the striatum, which leads to a reduced capacity for dopamine storage: levodopa arriving in the neuron is metabolized immediately to dopamine and released into the synapse. Postsynaptic factors may be at work, as shown by a rapidly waning response to apomorphine in fluctuating patients.

TABLE 7.2

Types of fluctuation

Long-duration motor fluctuations

- Dose-related early-morning worsening
- End–start dose failure (the drug fails to work sufficiently soon after administration, and/or its effects wear off before the next dose)
- 'On/off' fluctuations (see Table 7.3)
- Circadian or diurnal fluctuations (good response to levodopa in the morning but worsening response in the evening)
- Yo-yo movements (unpredictable)
- Postprandial worsening (following a high carbohydrate/protein meal)

Short-duration fluctuations (late in disease)

- Motor blocks, e.g. 'freezing' of gait: 'on/off' related/unpredictable
- Kinesia paradoxica (sudden relief from parkinsonism in response to stressful stimuli)

Unclassified fluctuations

- Premenstrual worsening (mechanism unclear)
- Late motor deterioration after prolonged levodopa withdrawal (up to 2 weeks later)
- Transient worsening after each dose of levodopa

TABLE 7.3

Factors underlying the development of motor fluctuations

Clinical symptoms	Possible causes
Wearing off	Presynaptic storage dysfunction
Delayed off	Delayed gastric emptying; intestinal absorption problems; possibly small-intestinal bacterial overgrowth
Dose-failure related (no 'on')	Delayed gastric emptying; intestinal absorbtion problems; blood–brain barrier
Random on–off	Striatal pharmacodynamic changes

Another factor is pharmacokinetic: plasma levels of levodopa become increasingly erratic due to variable absorption from the stomach and duodenum (involving some dietary interaction), together with a greater capacity for levodopa metabolism in the periphery. If low doses of combination therapy are used, decarboxylase may not be blocked effectively: carbidopa, 75 mg daily, is required. Of more importance is the peripheral O-methylation of dopa by catechol-O-methyl transferase (COMT) to 3-O-methyl-dopa, an inactive metabolite that does not cross the blood–brain barrier (see Figure 4.2).

Advanced disease. Fluctuations become increasingly unpredictable over a period of years and are difficult to relate to dopa dosage. 'Dose failures' may be related to poor absorption of levodopa or due to the recently described phenomenon of 'internalization' of dopamine receptors, so that drugs become ineffective for a period. Patients are significantly disabled and find it hard to plan their lives, not knowing whether they will be mobile ('on') or frozen ('off'). 'On/off' syndrome becomes the focus of their lives and is a challenging problem for clinicians (Table 7.4). Its appearance is related to the severity of disease and the underlying death of dopaminergic neurons.

"For family, friends and coworkers our on/offs can be scary. Like us, they wonder if our 'offs' will become a permanent state."

TABLE 7.4

Management strategies for fluctuations and dyskinesias

Type of fluctuation	Management
Suboptimal response at peak effect time/no 'on' period	• Increase levodopa dose • Add COMT inhibitor, e.g. entacapone • Add dopamine agonist
Early-morning dystonia	• Late-evening or night-time dose of controlled-release levodopa or long-acting dopamine agonist • Apomorphine injections • Botulinum toxin injection
'Wearing off'	• Shorten dosage interval • Pre-meal (up to 60 minutes) levodopa • Dispersible levodopa • COMT inhibitors • Dopamine agonist (short- or long-acting) • Controlled-release levodopa (best used before sleep) • MAOB inhibitors
Unpredictable 'on/off'	• Combination therapy with levodopa and dopamine agonist • Return to fewer doses of levodopa and combine with intermittent injections or continuous subcutaneous apomorphine, or intrajejunal infusion of levodopa • Dietary distribution of protein (small snacks and one large evening meal) • Deep brain stimulation
Freezing 'Off' related	• Increase dopaminergic therapy • Apomorphine (rescue injections)
Random or 'on' freezing	• Sensory cues
Anxiety related	• Anxiolytics, e.g. amitriptyline

CONTINUED

Timing of dyskinesia	Management
TABLE 7.4 (CONTINUED)	
Peak dose (usually choreic)	• Reduce individual levodopa dose
	• Frequent smaller doses, unchanged total
	• Addition of long-acting dopamine agonist with reduction in levodopa
	• Consider surgery
'Beginning' or 'end' dose	• Soluble levodopa before meals
	• COMT inhibitors
Diphasic dyskinesias	• Apomorphine infusion
	• Add cabergoline
	• Consider surgery

COMT, catechol-*O*-methyl transferase; MAOB, monoamine oxidase B.

Dyskinesias

Dyskinesias are hyperkinetic states mostly seen in patients with levodopa-treated Parkinson's disease. In the early stage of the disease, these states are often not noticed by patients and are a good sign of dopa responsiveness. A large body of research in animal models suggests that dyskinesias arise from alteration of dopaminergic tone in the denervated striatum, together with delivery of treatment by non-physiological pulsatile stimulation of dopamine receptors. This leads to cellular adaptations such as activation of transcription factors and alteration of downstream gene expression such as that of the immediate early genes.

Dyskinesias may be related to 'off' or 'on' periods, but as the disease advances they become a continuum and difficult to classify. 'Peak-dose' dyskinesias are the most common. They involve choreic or ballistic movements, and may be associated with a variety of non-motor symptoms such as pain, mood alterations and cognitive changes.

Dyskinesias may be socially unacceptable to carers, while patients may prefer to be dyskinetic when 'on'. Most dyskinesias progress and may lead to a reduced quality of life and weight loss. Reducing dopaminergic drugs will diminish dyskinesia, but may lead to a return of Parkinson's disease symptoms. Smaller doses of dopa given more frequently, or a combination of the drug with a dopamine agonist, may help, but problems are likely to reappear (see Table 7.4). The findings of a large number of preclinical and clinical studies indicate that continuous dopaminergic stimulation (CDS) may be the most desirable way to combat dyskinesias.

Dementia

Dementia is an important cause of comorbidity in parkinsonism; when cognition declines, mortality increases. Dementia is a bad sign and will often lead to the breakdown of support networks. Patients who are confused and hallucinating become difficult to manage at home and are frequently admitted to nursing homes. At this stage, life expectancy may be only 1–2 years.

Estimation of the incidence of dementia has proved difficult. Most parkinsonian patients have minor cognitive problems that are not apparent to spouses or relatives; 90% have deficits in frontal lobe tests, such as shifting sets (Wisconsin card sorting test). This reflects a rigidity of thought that may be apparent premorbidly for several years.

Characteristically, patients have difficulty 'changing their mind' and slowness of thought, with impairment of central reaction times. This can lead to a false estimation of cognitive function unless time is spent carefully assessing patients.

Global intellectual decline (dementia) is usually a feature of parkinsonism in the elderly, with more than 30% of patients over 70 years affected. Memory disturbance may be a warning sign, although younger patients may complain of short-term memory problems for many years. This may be due in part to drug therapy, particularly with anticholinergics, or to depression.

Hallucinosis is particularly worrying and often presages dementia (Table 7.5).

Excessive dopaminergic therapy or anticholinergic drugs can cause hallucinosis in the early stages of disease, but later hallucinosis may occur without drugs and is difficult to control. Often the next stage involves confusional episodes characterized by disorientation.

TABLE 7.5

Stages of hallucination in Parkinson's disease

Stage	Type
1	Vivid dreams (possibly predictive for development of florid hallucinations)
2	Preserved insight (seeing familial figures, deceased pets/ relatives)
3	Perceived as real (threatening/frightening visual hallucinations, rarely acoustic)

Dementia associated with Parkinson's disease has been termed subcortical, indicating predominant memory disorders, bradyphrenia and disorientation. This is in contrast to Alzheimer's disease, in which language difficulties and other cortical problems such as dyspraxia are predominant (Table 7.6). The distinction, however, is largely theoretical and is not substantiated by postmortem studies.

The cause of parkinsonian dementia is unclear. Autopsy studies have indicated a substantial contribution from Alzheimer-type pathology. Lewy bodies in the substantia nigra lead to a parkinsonian motor syndrome in life, and it is thought that they spread into the cortex and cause hallucinosis (occipital and temporal cortex) and other cognitive problems.

Diffuse Lewy body disease (now termed 'dementia with Lewy bodies', DLB) can present with parkinsonian characteristics, but cognitive decline and hallucinosis will be early features: 60% of Alzheimer's disease patients have extrapyramidal/parkinsonian signs in the later stages.

Management of dementia is difficult and requires the involvement of a multidisciplinary team (see *Fast Facts: Dementia*). The drug regimen used to treat Parkinson's disease should be kept as simple as possible, with the aim of achieving maximum mobility with minimum psychological disturbance (particularly hallucinosis). Anticholinergics, amantadine and even dopamine agonists may have to be stopped and the patient treated with the lowest possible dose of levodopa. Atypical antipsychotics such as quetiapine and clozapine may be employed in low dosages.

TABLE 7.6

Differences between parkinsonian dementia, dementia with Lewy bodies (DLB) and Alzheimer's disease

Feature	Parkinsonian dementia	DLB	Alzheimer's disease
Parkinsonian motor syndrome			
Presentation	Early	Late	Late
Disease course	Progressive	Progressive	Progressive
Response to levodopa	Sensitive	Waning response	No response
Dementia			
Presentation	Late	Early	Presenting feature
Features	Memory loss	Hallucinations	Memory loss
	Disorientation	Disorientation	Dysphasia
	Hallucinations	Memory loss	Dyspraxia, disorientation
Response to cholinergic therapy			
	Improvement	Possible behavioral changes	Helps memory for first year

Carers often prefer patients who are less mobile and less confused, because they are easier to care for. Wandering can be a problem; if confused, the patient will need constant supervision. Support for the carer is crucial in this situation and, if it cannot be provided, the patient will need residential care.

Depression and anxiety

Depression and anxiety are common accompaniments of Parkinson's disease ($\geq 50\%$, 2.7–70% depression, 50–66% anxiety), which may occur with the shock of the diagnosis or later on as a result of increasing disability. There is also evidence that depression is endogenous, intrinsic to the condition and part of the neurochemical profile.

Depression/anxiety is a marker for dementia in older patients. However, depression must not be mistaken for dementia. Pseudo-dementia can be mistaken for Parkinson's disease dementia. It is important to seek out depressive features and treat with antidepressants (tricyclic drugs or serotonin-reuptake inhibitors) if there is any suspicion of depression. The debate as to the advantages of the various antidepressants is ongoing (see *Fast Facts: Depression*).

Apathy

A syndrome of apathy distinct from depression, anxiety and fatigue is increasingly recognized in Parkinson's disease. Separate scales have been devised to assess apathy; it is important to recognize this syndrome, which may masquerade as depression.

Psychosis

Psychosis causes gross impairment in reality testing. Psychotic patients evaluate their perceptions abnormally, leading to incorrect interpretation of external reality. Psychosis consists of delusions (false beliefs about external reality) and hallucinations (sensory perceptions in the absence of external stimuli), and has a variety of causes (Table 7.7).

TABLE 7.7

Causes of psychosis in Parkinson's disease

- Dopaminergic drugs
- Dementia related to Parkinson's disease
- Development of dementia with Lewy bodies
- Toxic confusional state in Parkinson's disease induced by:
  - infection (particularly urinary or upper respiratory tract infection)
  - metabolic/endocrine upset (e.g. diabetic ketoacidosis)
  - malnutrition
  - dehydration
  - sudden withdrawal of dopaminergic drugs or amantadine

Drug-induced psychosis appears to result from altered function within dopamine projection neurons originating in the ventral tegmental area. Overstimulation of mesencephalic–limbic dopamine receptors causes limbic system dysfunction, leading to psychosis. The management of drug-induced psychosis is outlined in Figure 7.2.

Typical antipsychotic drugs (e.g. haloperidol, chlorpromazine) antagonize dopamine D_2 receptors and may cause extrapyramidal side effects such as tardive dyskinesias and parkinsonism. Atypical antipsychotics (e.g. quetiapine, clozapine) appear to control psychosis without significantly compromising motor function and so are more suitable for treating psychosis in Parkinson's disease (Table 7.8). These agents bind more selectively to serotonin and mesolimbic dopamine receptors than they do to striatal dopamine receptors. However, olanzapine should be avoided as it may significantly worsen Parkinson's disease even in small doses. Ondansetron, an antiemetic with action at the serotonin receptors, is also useful in some cases.

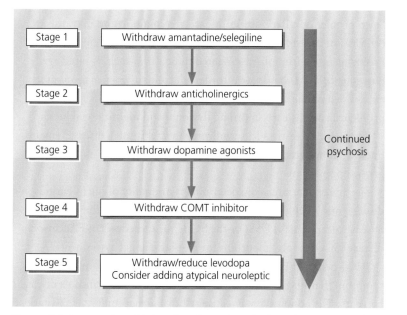

Figure 7.2 Strategy for withdrawing dopaminergic drugs in patients with drug-induced psychosis. COMT, catechol-*O*-methyl transferase.

TABLE 7.8

Features of atypical antipsychotic (neuroleptic) drug treatment in Parkinson's disease

- All should be started at very low doses
- Drowsiness is common because of antihistamine and antiserotonergic action
- Anticholinergics should be withdrawn before use, otherwise delirium may be precipitated
- Quetiapine is the drug of choice in most cases
- White blood cell count is mandatory with clozapine (weekly)
- Ondansetron (a novel 5-HT$_3$ antagonist with a potent antiemetic effect) is expensive and may be occasionally useful
- Postural hypotension is a common side effect
- If an atypical neuroleptic, e.g. sulpiride, is used, a compensatory increase in levodopa dose may be required

Sleep disorders

Sleep problems in Parkinson's disease are common and may affect 60–98% of individuals at both early and late stages of the disease. Problems range from disease-related difficulties, such as rapid eye movement (REM) behavior disorder, sleep-maintenance insomnia, excessive daytime sleepiness and nocturia, to possibly drug-related problems, such as early-morning dystonia and night-time akinesia.

The cause of restless legs syndrome in Parkinson's disease remains unclear, although it occurs around twice as commonly as in the general population.

Sleep problems are a key determinant of quality of life in Parkinson's disease, and sleep scales specific to the disease such as the Parkinson's Disease Sleep Scale (PDSS) or the SCale for Outcomes in PArkinson's disease (SCOPA) are important for regular clinical assessments.

REM behavior disorder in particular has emerged as an important symptom that may predict the motor diagnosis of Parkinson's disease by years. The condition may cause self or partner injury, as the patient tends to act out violent dreams in REM sleep. The pathophysiology may involve brainstem nuclei, such as the pedunculopontine nucleus and locus ceruleus, which are involved in stage 2 disease (by Braak staging; see pages 20–1; Figure 2.3), with a motor diagnosis being made in stage 3.

Autonomic problems

Autonomic problems occur with increasing frequency in advanced disease, as has been shown in the Non-Motor Symptoms Questionnaire (NMSQuest) study. The problems include gastrointestinal symptoms (constipation, dribbling, dysphagia), orthostatic hypotension, excessive sweating or hyperhidrosis, bladder dysfunction such as detrusor muscle hyperactivity, and sexual dysfunction.

Sensory problems

Sensory problems associated with the disease mainly comprise pain syndromes and akathisia, usually in the 'off' state. Pain is a key unmet need in Parkinson's disease and can be of several types. The King's Parkinson's pain scale (KPP) has recently been validated as the first

---

Key points – long-term complications

- Virtually all patients taking prolonged levodopa experience long-term complications within 2–3 years of treatment.
- Most dyskinesias progress; smaller, more frequent doses of levodopa, or a combination of the drug with a dopamine agonist, may help but problems are likely to reappear.
- Depression should be treated with antidepressants; depression/ anxiety is a marker for dementia in older patients.
- Patients who are confused and hallucinating become difficult to manage at home and life expectancy may diminish to 1–2 years.
- Sleep disorders may affect 60–98% of patients with Parkinson's disease; the presence of rapid eye movement (REM) behavior disorder may precede the motor diagnosis by years.
- The cause of death in Parkinson's disease is most commonly a secondary comorbid disorder.

pain scale for Parkinson's disease; it allows classification of different types of pain in Parkinson's disease and can be used to devise targeted treatment strategies.

Declaration of non-motor symptoms

Early recognition of non-motor symptoms is important, as studies show that the burden of non-motor symptoms as a whole is the key determinant to quality of life. An international study showed that large numbers of patients do not declare these symptoms unless specifically asked. This can lead to a shocking neglect of symptoms that may be treatable, even in well-established centers of Parkinson's disease care.

The NMSQuest (see Figure 3.5) empowers patients to declare their non-motor symptoms to health professionals (see Figure 3.6).

Key references

Aarsland D, Andersen K, Larsen JP et al. The rate of cognitive decline in Parkinson disease. *Arch Neurol* 2004;61:1906–11.

Chaudhuri KR, Martinez-Martin P, Schapira AH et al. International multicenter pilot study of the first comprehensive self-completed nonmotor symptoms questionnaire for Parkinson's disease: the NMSQuest study. *Mov Disord* 2006;21:916–23.

Chaudhuri KR, Prieto-Jurcynska C, Naidu Y et al. The nondeclaration of nonmotor symptoms of Parkinson's disease to health care professionals: an international study using the nonmotor symptoms questionnaire. *Mov Disord* 2010;25:697–701.

Emre M. Dementia associated with Parkinson's disease. *Lancet Neurol* 2003;2:229–37.

Haddad M, Gunn J. *Fast Facts: Depression*, 3rd edn. Oxford: Health Press, 2011.

Marsden CD, Parkes JD. 'On-off' effects in patients with Parkinson's disease on chronic levodopa therapy. *Lancet* 1976;1:292–6.

Playfer JR, Hindle JV, eds. *Parkinson's Disease in the Older Patient*. London: Arnold, 2001: 215–38.

Sato K, Hatano T, Yamashiro K et al. Prognosis of Parkinson's disease: time to stage III, IV, V, and to motor fluctuations. *Mov Disord* 2006;21:1384–95.

Tanner CM, Aston DA. Epidemiology of Parkinson's disease and akinetic syndromes. *Curr Opin Neurol* 2000;13:427–30.

Whalley LJ, Breitner JCS. *Fast Facts: Dementia*, 2nd edn. Oxford: Health Press, 2009.

A variety of etiologies that are not secondary to the idiopathic loss of neurons in the substantia nigra may cause parkinsonian syndromes; they include infections, drugs, toxins and structural lesions. In addition, there are a number of degenerative diseases that have a more complex clinical picture than Parkinson's disease and a poorer response to therapy (Table 8.1). It may be impossible to distinguish idiopathic Parkinson's disease from other parkinsonian syndromes by clinical features alone.

An extensive review of the patient's medical history and diagnostic tests, such as neuroimaging, can aid diagnosis (see Chapter 3).

Drug-induced parkinsonism

This is the most common cause of secondary parkinsonism and it is often misdiagnosed as Parkinson's disease, because clinical features may be indistinguishable. It causes rigidity, bradykinesia, tremor and gait disturbance, and may be asymmetric. Although several medications are associated with secondary parkinsonism (Table 8.2), dopamine-blocking agents (neuroleptics) such as prochlorperazine or chlorpromazine are the most common offending agents, and are often prescribed to the elderly for non-specific complaints such as dizziness. The incidence of drug-induced parkinsonism is estimated to be 15–40% in patients receiving neuroleptics, and its prevalence increases with age.

There is some evidence that patients who develop drug-induced parkinsonism may have subclinical Lewy body Parkinson's disease, which may be unmasked by dopamine-blocking agents.

The effects of dopamine-blocking agents may be prolonged, and drug-induced parkinsonism may take up to 9 months to disappear. Treatment consists of withdrawal of the offending medication. If drug withdrawal is impractical, patients are given the lowest possible dose or are changed to a new atypical agent, such as clozapine or quetiapine. Anticholinergics may be beneficial; levodopa treatment has not been studied systematically.

TABLE 8.1

Degenerative parkinsonian syndromes

- Corticobasal ganglionic degeneration
- Dementia with Lewy bodies
- Multiple system atrophy (MSA)
  - MSA-P (predominance of parkinsonian features)
  - MSA-C (predominance of cerebellar features)
- Progressive supranuclear palsy
- Hereditary degenerative diseases
- Autosomal-dominant cerebellar ataxias
  - Machado–Joseph disease, also called spinocerebellar ataxia type 3 (SCA-3)
- Neuronal brain iron accumulation syndromes
  - pantothenate kinase-associated neurodegeneration (PKAN) (*PANK2* mutation)
  - phospholipase A2-associated neurodegeneration (PLAN) (*PLA2G6* mutation)
  - fatty acid hydroxylase-associated neurodegeneration (FAHN) (*FA2H* mutation)
  - neuroferritinopathy
  - mutations in *FTL* encoding L-ferritin
  - aceruloplasminemia
  - static enchephalopathy of childhood with neurodegeneration in adulthood (SENDA) syndrome
  - Kufor–Rakeb disease (*PARK9* mutation)
- Prion disorders
- Hereditary frontotemporal dementias
- Huntington's disease
- Neuroacanthocytosis
- Wilson's disease
- Whipple's disease
- X-linked dystonia–parkinsonism (Lubag)
- Parkinsonism–dementia–amyotrophic lateral sclerosis complex of Guam (an atypical unclassifiable parkinsonism found in people on Guadeloupe)

TABLE 8.2

Drugs that can induce parkinsonism

Inhibitors of dopamine synthesis or precursors of a false neurotransmitter

- α-methyl-paratyrosine
- α-methyldopa

Inhibitors of presynaptic dopamine storage

- Reserpine
- Tetrabenazine

Blockers of postsynaptic D_2 receptors

Neuroleptics

- Phenothiazines
  - prochlorperazine
  - amitriptyline
  - thioridazine
  - promethazine
  - fluphenazine
  - mesoridazine
  - trifluoperazine
  - chlorpromazine
  - thiethylperazine
  - perphenazine
- Butyrophenones
  - haloperidol

- Thioxanthenes
  - thiothixene
- Benzamides
  - metoclopramide
- Dihydroindolone
  - molindone
- Dibenzoxazepine
  - loxapine

Miscellaneous D_2-blocking agents

- Tetrabenazine
- Flunarizine
- Amoxapine

γ-aminobutyric acid agonists

- Sodium valproate

Calcium-channel blockers

- Cinnarizine

Progressive supranuclear palsy

Progressive supranuclear palsy (PSP; Steele–Richardson–Olszewski syndrome) presents with gait disturbance and falls (predominantly backward) in over 50% of cases, and is a disease of later life. The pathological hallmark is tau protein-positive filamentous inclusions, known as neurofibrillary tangles, in the glia and neurons.

The clinical picture consists of supranuclear gaze palsy, particularly down-gaze with nuchal extension, and predominant truncal extensor rigidity. Varying degrees of bradykinesia, dysphagia, personality changes and other behavioral disturbances, such as a subcortical frontal dementia, coexist.

Eye-movement abnormalities (external ocular movements) are very characteristic but may not be present at disease onset. However, patients rarely die without developing these abnormalities. The external ocular movements consist of square-wave jerks, instability of fixation, slow or hypometric saccades and predominantly down-gaze supranuclear palsy. Most simply, patients are unable to look up or down to command, but vertical eye movements following a target are preserved early on, and vestibulo-ocular reflex is retained until very late.

Limb rest-tremor is rare but has been reported. The presence of asymmetric signs, in particular rest-tremor, would favor a diagnosis of Parkinson's disease over PSP.

Variants of PSP include progressive dementia resembling Alzheimer's disease, pure akinesia and a parkinsonian phenotype. PSP can be confused with frontotemporal dementia, corticobasal degeneration or Pick's disease. Sophisticated MRI of the brain can distinguish PSP from Parkinson's disease, in that the midbrain tectum and tegmentum atrophy in advanced PSP; in addition, the course of PSP is progressive without significant response to levodopa.

Usually, patients die within 5–10 years because of increasing bulbar problems and immobility.

Pathologically confirmed PSP has been shown to have two clinical phenotypes: Richardson's syndrome and PSP-parkinsonism (PSP-P). Richardson's syndrome makes up the majority of cases, and is characterized by the early onset of postural instability and falls, supranuclear vertical gaze palsy and cognitive dysfunction. However,

PSP-P is characterized by an asymmetric onset, tremor and a moderate initial therapeutic response to levodopa, and the condition is frequently confused with Parkinson's disease. Patients with PSP-P may develop the other features of PSP described above later in the course of the disease.

Multiple system atrophy

Multiple system atrophy (MSA) consists of a variable combination of parkinsonism with autonomic, pyramidal or cerebellar symptoms and signs. In the past, patients were categorized as having striatonigral type (SND) if parkinsonian signs were dominant, olivopontocerebellar type (OPCA) if cerebellar signs predominated and Shy–Drager syndrome if autonomic signs were dominant.

Criteria for the diagnosis of MSA were formulated by Quinn in 1989 and 1994 and subsequently by Gilman et al. in 1998. The SND and OPCA variants are now called MSA-P and MSA-C, respectively (see Table 8.1), and the use of the term Shy–Drager syndrome is discouraged. The pathological feature of MSA is the glial cytoplasmic inclusions that stain positive for α-synuclein.

The main problem is in differentiating Parkinson's disease from the striatonigral type in which the parkinsonian features of MSA include progressive bradykinesia, rigidity and postural instability, and signs that are usually bilateral. Useful clinical clues include disproportionate anterocollis, truncal dystonia (Pisa syndrome), characteristic sighing and the presence of cold, blue hands. Autonomic failure occurs early in MSA and is more severe than in idiopathic Parkinson's disease.

The response to levodopa is commonly incomplete and benefit usually declines within 1–2 years of treatment.

Urinary symptoms are very common. Urodynamic testing reveals a combination of detrusor hyperreflexia and urethral sphincter weakness, which occur in other conditions such as PSP. Neuroimaging may reveal hypointensity of the putamen or an abnormal cross sign, known as the 'hot cross bun' sign, in the pons. However, studies suggest that a considerable number of people who are diagnosed with MSA or PSP turn out to have an alternative histopathological diagnosis on postmortem analysis.

Dementia with Lewy bodies

In dementia with Lewy bodies (DLB), widespread areas of neocortex as well as brainstem and diencephalic neurons have Lewy bodies. Some patients may have associated neurofibrillary tangles consistent with coincidental Alzheimer's disease.

Parkinsonian DLB may be indistinguishable from Parkinson's disease, but patients with the former have early-onset dementia (progressive cognitive decline interfering with normal social and occupational function) and may have hallucinations, delusions and even psychosis in the absence of dopaminergic therapy.

Clinical criteria for diagnosis were developed in 1996 and updated in 1999. Core features of DLB include fluctuations in cognition and attention, recurrent and persistent visual hallucinations and parkinsonian motor signs. Repeated and early falls and neuroleptic sensitivity can be seen. Rarely, patients develop supranuclear gaze palsy; this may lead to the condition being mistaken for PSP.

Response to levodopa tends not to be as complete as in Parkinson's disease, although some patients do respond. The electroencephalogram recording in DLB may be abnormal with background posterior slowing and frontally dominant burst activity, which is not a feature of Parkinson's disease.

Corticobasal ganglionic degeneration

Corticobasal ganglionic degeneration (CBGD), also known as corticodentato-nigral degeneration with neuronal achromasia, typically presents in the sixth or seventh decade with slowly progressive, unilateral development of tremor, apraxia and rigidity in an upper limb.

The condition is characterized by progressive gait disturbances, cortical sensory loss and stimulus-sensitive myoclonus that results in a jerky useless hand. A jerky useless lower extremity is uncommon, but may occur. The phenomenon is known as the alien limb and can occur in about 50% of patients. Gait disturbance consists of a slightly wide-based, apraxic gait rather than the typical festinating gait of Parkinson's disease. Patients with CBGD do not benefit from levodopa, and the disease course is relentlessly progressive.

The clinical spectrum of this disorder has been expanded to include early-onset dementia and aphasia. Other clinical signs include frontotemporal dementia, and visuospatial and visuoperceptive deficits. MRI reveals focal atrophy, particularly in the parietal areas, and positron emission tomography (PET) scans show an asymmetric decrease in regional cerebral glucose metabolic rates.

Parkinsonism in young adults

The onset of parkinsonism before the age of 40 years is usually called young-onset parkinsonism. Onset of Parkinson's disease at this age is not rare. When symptoms begin before the age of 20, the term juvenile parkinsonism may be used. Parkinsonism at this early age typically occurs as a component of a more widespread degenerative disorder or a genetic disorder.

Disorders such as Wilson's disease, Huntington's disease and dentatorubral-pallidoluysian atrophy should be ruled out by appropriate copper measurements and genetic testing. Often, young-onset Parkinson's disease can remain exquisitely sensitive to levodopa for many years, with concurrent development of increasing dyskinesia. The earlier the onset of Parkinson's disease, the more likely that genetic factors are important, and the greater the need for enquiry into family history.

Dopa-responsive dystonia. Patients with young-onset parkinsonism manifest dystonia, which may respond to dopaminergic drugs. However, there is another entity called dopa-responsive dystonia (Segawa's disease), which usually starts in childhood or adolescence. Dystonia is the predominant phenotypic expression; autosomal dominance is the usual inheritance. Patients have a guanosine triphosphate (GTP)-cyclohydrolase deficiency, the genetic abnormality for which is found on chromosome 14.

The disorder characteristically shows marked diurnal variation, and may start in childhood with an unusual gait. Patients demonstrate an excellent and sustained response to low-dose levodopa. Childhood dystonia or unexplained spastic gait should therefore be given a trial of low-dose levodopa, 100 mg once daily. Some family members may show later-onset parkinsonism.

PET scans demonstrate markedly reduced 6-fluorodopa uptake in patients with young-onset Parkinson's disease, while fluorodopa uptake is normal in patients with dopa-responsive dystonia.

Wilson's disease should be considered in every case of young-onset parkinsonism, because it is treatable and the consequences of non-recognition can be grievous. The most common neurological manifestations include tremor, dystonia, rigidity, dysarthria, drooling and ataxia. A combination of parkinsonism and ataxia is characteristic of neurological Wilson's disease. Tremor typically involves the upper limbs and the head, and rarely the lower limbs; classically, the tremor is coarse, irregular and present during action. Holding the arms forward and flexed horizontally may demonstrate the activity of the proximal muscles (wing-beating tremor).

Kayser–Fleischer rings – rings of brownish-green pigmentation – due to copper deposition in the cornea may be easy to recognize in patients with light-colored irises, and are best appreciated with a careful slit-lamp examination performed by an ophthalmologist.

Almost all patients with neurological features have MRI abnormalities in the basal ganglia. There is a pattern of symmetric bilateral concentric-laminar T2 hyperintensity in the putamen and involvement of the pars compacta of the substantia nigra, periaqueductal gray matter, the pontine tegmentum and the thalamus.

The most useful diagnostic test results are a low serum ceruloplasmin level and a raised 24-hour urinary copper excretion. Slit-lamp examination should be performed looking for Kayser–Fleischer rings (see above). Not all patients have a low ceruloplasmin level because inflammation, infection or oral contraceptive use may cause false elevations. Liver biopsy to show copper deposition remains the gold standard diagnostic test.

Juvenile Huntington's disease is an autosomal-dominant neurodegenerative disorder that typically presents with chorea, difficulty with gait and cognitive problems. However, the Westphal variant of the disease, which affects the young, may resemble parkinsonism.

Eye-movement abnormalities, including apraxia, distinguish juvenile Huntington's disease from Parkinson's disease.

Gene testing for Huntington's disease (which may show a cytosine, adenine and guanine [CAG] repeat or 'expansion' greater than 35 trinucleotides) should be performed in all patients with juvenile-onset Parkinson's disease, and in adults with unusual features and cognitive decline.

Hemiparkinsonism hemiatrophy syndrome

Patients with this syndrome have a long-standing hemiatrophy of the body and develop a progressive bradykinesia with dystonic movements around the age of 40 years. Ipsilateral corticospinal tract signs, which are not a feature of Parkinson's disease, may be found. Neuroimaging reveals atrophy of the contralateral hemisphere with compensatory ventricular dilatation.

Neuroacanthocytosis

Neuroacanthocytosis is a rare cause of parkinsonism and typically presents with a hyperkinetic movement disorder, including chorea, tic-like features and polyneuropathy. MRI shows characteristic atrophy of the caudate nucleus and hyperintensity in the putamen on T2-weighted images. Acanthocytes are revealed on a fresh blood smear.

Secondary parkinsonism

The term 'secondary parkinsonism' refers to parkinsonism induced by known agents or factors. In addition to drugs (see page 139; Table 8.2), these include infections, toxins, structural lesions and vascular disease.

Encephalitis lethargica and postencephalitic parkinsonism. From 1919 to 1926 there were several pandemic outbreaks of encephalitis lethargica (von Economo's encephalitis). Patients had headache, fever, somnolence and ophthalmoplegia. After a variable delay, a number of patients developed parkinsonism associated with psychiatric abnormalities, ophthalmoplegia and oculogyric crises. In this

147

condition, tremor tends to be less prominent than in Parkinson's disease, and other movement disorders, including dystonia, may be seen. The oculogyric crises, which do not occur in idiopathic Parkinson's disease, are characterized by forceful deviation of the eyes, usually upwards or upwards and laterally. Sometimes obsessional thoughts or fear and anxiety accompany attacks.

Parkinsonism is rarely associated with other forms of viral encephalitis, such as the arboviruses, measles, polio, coxsackie, echoviruses, herpes simplex, varicella, Japanese encephalitis or western equine encephalitis.

The response of postencephalitic parkinsonism to levodopa is inconsistent and may wane after an excellent improvement or 'awakening'. In a follow-up study of 50 patients, a third continued to benefit, a third showed no response and the remaining patients could not tolerate the drug.

Other infectious etiologies. Neurological complications, including parkinsonism, may occur in patients with AIDS. Parkinsonian features may be secondary to AIDS-associated cerebral infections or cerebral infection with HIV alone. Other rare infections have been reported to cause parkinsonism, including fungal infections, *Mycoplasma pneumoniae*, syphilis, Creutzfeldt–Jakob disease, and cryptococcal and cysticercus infections. In this situation it is usually obvious that parkinsonism is part of a more widespread brain disorder and/or there is evidence of central-nervous-system infection (fever, meningism, confusion).

Toxins. Parkinsonism can be caused by a variety of toxins including carbon monoxide, 1-methyl-4-phenyl-1,2,3,6-tetrahydropyridine (MPTP) (Figure 8.1), manganese and cyanide. Manganism is a neurological syndrome caused by excessive exposure to high levels of manganese. The clinical features include parkinsonism characterized by early difficulties with gait and balance, early speech problems, and dystonia involving the face (grimace) and feet (cock walk). In general, rest-tremor is absent and the clinical features are symmetric. In addition, response to levodopa is poor or non-existent. The

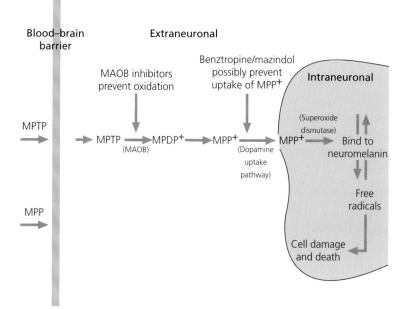

Blood–brain barrier

Extraneuronal

MAOB inhibitors prevent oxidation

Benztropine/mazindol possibly prevent uptake of MPP⁺

Intraneuronal

MPTP →

→ MPTP $\xrightarrow{\text{(MAOB)}}$ MPDP⁺ → MPP⁺ $\xrightarrow{\text{(Dopamine uptake pathway)}}$ MPP⁺ → Bind to neuromelanin

(Superoxide dismutase)

MPP →

Free radicals

Cell damage and death

Figure 8.1 The mechanism of action of 1-methyl-4-phenyl-1,2,3,6-tetrahydropyridine (MPTP) and how it causes parkinsonism. MAOB, monoamine oxidase B; MPDP, 1-methyl-4-phenyl-2,3-dihydropyridine; MPP, 1-methyl-4-phenylpyridine.

characteristic imaging features are a bilateral symmetric hyperintensity on T1-weighted MRI in the globus pallidi, and an intact nigrostriatal dopaminergic pathway on imaging of the dopaminergic system. The pathology of manganism involves the globus pallidus and to a lesser extent the putamen, with sparing of the substantia nigra zona compacta. The clinical, imaging and therapeutic features have been described in well-defined groups who have been occupationally exposed to high levels of manganese (e.g. manganese smelters, manganese ore crushers), as well as in patients with liver failure and those receiving total parenteral nutrition. More recently, an outbreak of manganism was reported in individuals abusing an illicit drug made with a compound that contained manganese. The role of manganese in welding fumes in relation to Parkinson's disease is controversial (see page 31) and is being investigated.

MPTP causes a pure motor parkinsonian syndrome that responds well to levodopa. Other toxins produce a more complex parkinsonian syndrome unresponsive to levodopa.

Structural lesions that either directly or indirectly affect the basal ganglia may produce parkinsonism. Lesions secondary to hypoxia, hydrocephalus, tumors, vascular disease including strokes and vascular malformations, and demyelinating lesions have been associated with parkinsonism. These are almost always identified on MRI scans.

Hydrocephalus. Patients with hydrocephalus may develop parkinsonian symptoms months or years after initially presenting with hydrocephalus (Figure 8.2), or parkinsonism may develop acutely because of shunt failure, with resolution following shunt revision. Clinically, patients may have tremor, rigidity and bradykinesia.

Normal-pressure hydrocephalus is characterized by the triad of gait difficulty, dementia and urinary incontinence. Poor postural reflexes and flexed posture may also be seen. The hydrocephalus should be treated either by shunting or by shunt revision in the case of malfunction. If parkinsonian symptoms do not respond to shunting, some patients may be sensitive to dopaminergic therapy with a

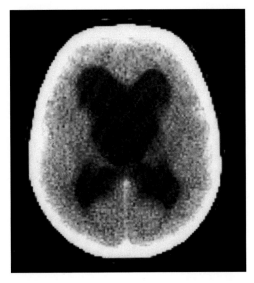

Figure 8.2 Scan of hydrocephalic brain, showing massive dilatation of the cerebral ventricles.

dopamine agonist or levodopa. Normal-pressure hydrocephalus is diagnosed frequently, and many patients undergo shunting without adequate results. This may reflect difficulty in selecting patients who will benefit from treatment: those presenting with gait difficulty alone show the best response, while those with a predominantly cognitive presentation respond poorly and may have a neurodegenerative problem such as Alzheimer's disease.

Tumors are a rare cause of parkinsonism. Those associated with parkinsonism occur in several regions of the brain including the striatum, frontal lobe, temporal lobe, parietal lobe, thalamus/ hypothalamus, substantia nigra, midbrain and third ventricle. A variety of tumor types have been described, including:

- glioma
- meningioma
- lymphoma
- fibrosarcoma
- metastasis.

Usually patients present with a one-sided, progressive syndrome that does not respond to levodopa. Other signs, such as upper motor neuron signs and a rapidly progressive disease course, will distinguish tumor-related parkinsonism from Parkinson's disease and will determine whether a diagnostic scan is necessary.

Vascular disease is a rare cause of a straightforward parkinsonian syndrome with a variety of clinical presentations. Onset is either acute or subacute, and symptoms (usually bilateral) are those seen in classic Parkinson's disease, including tremor, bradykinesia, rigidity and postural instability. The disease course may be stable from onset or progressive, or may resolve spontaneously. A subgroup of patients may present with predominant lower-extremity symptoms, such as a gait disturbance with minimal upper-extremity symptoms (lower-body parkinsonism), or walking with small steps (marche à petits pas), which is characteristic of vascular disease. Often, additional signs such as spasticity or abnormal plantar reflexes are present.

Post-traumatic parkinsonism. An isolated head injury seldom leads to parkinsonism unless it causes significant brain damage. However, multiple minor head injuries may cause cumulative damage resulting in parkinsonism and dementia, as seen in boxers who have had multiple knock-outs (dementia pugilistica). Radiologically, diffuse brain atrophy and a large cavum septum pellucidum, a cavity within the dividing membranes of the lateral ventricles, characterize this condition.

Miscellaneous causes. Parkinsonism may occur transiently during alcohol withdrawal. Metabolic causes include hypoparathyroidism with basal ganglia calcifications. There are a few reports of Sjögren's syndrome with associated parkinsonism, but whether parkinsonism is more common in Sjögren's syndrome or the association is coincidental is unclear. Parkinsonian features have been described in central pontine and extrapontine myelinolysis, and in Behçet's disease.

Key points – other parkinsonian syndromes

- It may be impossible to distinguish Parkinson's disease from other parkinsonian syndromes by clinial features alone.
- Progressive supranuclear palsy presents with gait disturbance and falls in later life; asymmetric signs (e.g. rest-tremor) favor a diagnosis of Parkinson's disease.
- Patients with parkinsonian dementia with Lewy bodies have early-onset dementia, and may have hallucinations or psychosis in the absence of dopaminergic therapy.
- Parkinsonism that presents before the age of 20 is more likely to be the result of a widespread degenerative or genetic disorder.
- Drug-induced parkinsonism is the most common cause of secondary parkinsonism.

Key references

Cummings JL. Reconsidering diagnostic criteria for dementia with Lewy bodies. Highlights from the Third International Workshop on Dementia with Lewy Bodies and Parkinson's Disease Dementia, September 17–20, 2003, Newcastle Upon Tyne, United Kingdom. *Rev Neurol Dis* 2004;1:31–4.

Gilman S, Low PA, Quinn N et al. Consensus statement on the diagnosis of multiple system atrophy. American Autonomic Society and American Academy of Neurology. *Clin Auton Res* 1998;8:359–62.

Hughes AJ, Daniel SE, Ben-Shlomo Y, Lees AJ. The accuracy of diagnosis of parkinsonian syndromes in a specialist movement disorder service. *Brain* 2002;125:861–70.

McKeith IG, Galasko D, Kosaka K et al. Consensus guidelines for the clinical and pathologic diagnosis of dementia with Lewy bodies (DLB): report of the consortium on DLB international workshop. *Neurology* 1996;47:1113–24.

McKeith I, Mintzer J, Aarsland D et al; International Psychogeriatric Association Expert Meeting on DLB. Dementia with Lewy Bodies. *Lancet Neurol* 2004;3:19–28.

Quinn N. Multiple system atrophy – the nature of the beast. *J Neurol Neurosurg Psychiatry* 1989;suppl: 78–89.

Steele JC. Progressive supranuclear palsy. *Brain* 1972;95:693–704.

Wenning GK, Poewe W, eds. Atypical parkinsonian disorders. *Mov Disord* 2005;20(suppl 12): S1–126.

153

Although research has helped to develop a range of pharmacological and surgical therapies for Parkinson's disease, we are still unable to cure the disease or slow its progression. In future, the goal of treatment will be prevention and cure, and management strategies will be based on finding a treatable cause (Table 9.1).

TABLE 9.1

Areas of investigation for pharmacological treatment

Restoration of dopamine

- Dopamine creation
- Dopamine conservation
- Selective striatal dopamine-receptor stimulation

Non-dopaminergic modulation

- Newer anticholinergics
- Adenosine A$_2$ antagonists
- Cannabinoids
- α-adrenoceptor antagonists

Neuroprotective therapy (to slow, halt or reverse progressive neurodegeneration)

- Antiglutamate agents (*N*-methyl-D-aspartate antagonists), e.g. riluzole, remacemide, amantadine, modafinil, memantine
- Antioxidants, e.g. ascorbic acid, vitamin E, rasagiline
- Antiapoptosis agents, e.g. selegiline, dopamine agonists, TCH-346, CEP-1347
- Mitochondrial enhancers, e.g. coenzyme Q10, creatine
- Anti-inflammatory drugs, e.g. cyclooxygenase (COX-1, COX-2) inhibitors, minocycline
- Trophic factors, e.g. glial-cell-line-derived neurotrophic factor, GPI-1485, GM-1 ganglioside
- Protein aggregate inhibitors, e.g. radicicola, sirolimus (rapamycin), trehalose, small ubiquitin-like modifier (SUMO)-1, valproic acid

Evidence suggests that the neurodegenerative process in Parkinson's disease is a final outcome of several interrelated processes:
- oxidative stress from toxic free-radical production
- mitochondrial dysfunction
- accumulation of excitotoxic molecules, such as nitric oxide and oxidative free radicals
- inflammatory changes.

A combination of these processes results in cell death by both necrosis and apoptosis. These depend on external (environmental) and internal (genetic) factors, the balance of which varies from patient to patient.

New medicines in development

Dopaminergic treatment. Several compounds are being developed that continue to exploit the dopamine pathway (Table 9.2), but selectively stimulate different dopamine receptors (D_1–D_5). Some compounds, such as ABT-431, are thought to selectively stimulate dopamine D_1 rather than D_2 receptors. Others, such as U-95667E, stimulate D_2 receptors selectively. Preferential stimulation of dopamine receptors may offer control of parkinsonism without dyskinesia, particularly as there is some evidence to show that D_1 action is beneficial for bladder function in patients with Parkinson's disease, while D_3 selectivity may increase the risk of impulse control disorders.

Neuroprotection remains a key therapeutic target and various strategies are being investigated, including the use of antioxidants, enhancers of mitochondrial function, antiapoptotic agents, glutamate antagonists, anti-inflammatory drugs and antiprotein aggregation drugs (see Tables 9.1 and 9.3).

Glutamate, an excitatory amino acid, may lead to overstimulation and cell death in the substantia nigra, so compounds that block glutamate stimulation via N-methyl-D-aspartate receptors are under investigation. Riluzole, a glutamate antagonist, was investigated for potential neuroprotective effect in untreated patients, but this trial was stopped because interim analysis showed no effect on disease progression. Remacemide, another proposed neuroprotective agent, has also failed to demonstrate any significant beneficial effect in

TABLE 9.2

New dopaminergic treatment in development

Drug	Route of delivery	Action
New methods of delivering levodopa		
ND0612/ND0611	Subcutaneous	Continuous infusion of LD-CD
XP21279	Oral	Prodrug – ER LD
AP LD-CD (The Accordion pill)	Oral	Prolongs gastric retention
CVT-301	Inhalation	Dry powder aerosol
Inhibition of catechol-O-methyltransferase (COMT)		
Opicapone (BIA 9-1067)	Oral o.d.	Inhibition of COMT enzyme
ODM-101 LD-CD-entacapone)	Oral	Optimized combination of levodopa plus inhibition of dopa-decarboxylase and COMT
New dopamine agonists		
APL 130277 (apomorphine)	Sublingual	Delivers apomorphine by thin-strip film
VR 010 (apomorphine)	Inhalation	Delivers apomorphine by inhalator device

CD, carbidopa; ER, extended release; LD, levodopa; o.d., once daily.

preliminary clinical trials. Modafinil, used for treating sleepiness, is another drug with antiglutamate action that is under consideration.

A pilot study (referred to as QE2) investigating a possible disease-altering effect of coenzyme Q10 (a fat-soluble vitamin) in a small number of patients with Parkinson's disease suggested a possible beneficial effect at a large dose (1200 mg/day). These results are being studied in a larger trial (QE3). However, the findings of the Neuroprotection Exploratory Trials in Parkinson's Disease (NET-PD),

TABLE 9.3

Potential neuroprotective strategies in Parkinson's disease

Agent	Mode of action
Isradipine	Calcium channel antagonist
Exenatide	GLP-1 antagonist
Ambroxol	Secretolytic, anti-inflammatory
α-synuclein vaccination	Reduces α-synuclein levels; active/passive immunization
CERE-120	Neurotrophic gene therapy
Inosine	Antixoxidant
Deferiprone	Antixoxidant
Intraputaminal GDNF	Neurotrophic factor
GM1 ganglioside	Neurotrophic factor
Pioglitazone	Peroxisome proliferator-activated receptor-γ agonist

GDNF, glial cell-line-derived neurotrophic factor; GLP-1, glucagon-like peptide 1; GM1, monosialotetrahexosyl (ganglioside).

run by the US National Institutes of Health to find drugs with the potential to slow the progression of the disease, were discouraging for this compound as it was not considered to be any better than placebo.

Apoptosis causes cell death, and antiapoptotic agents such as TCH-346 and caspase inhibitors have been evaluated and found to be ineffective in slowing down the course of Parkinson's disease. Minocycline, a caspase inhibitor, has been investigated in a NET-PD trial and is not going to be studied any further.

Free-radical production may cause dopamine neuronal degeneration. All of the following may help prevent cell death: 'spin-trap' agents that reduce oxidative stress by scavenging free radicals; agents that chelate iron, such as some forms of apomorphine; or agents that enhance glutathione release. Examples are CU 02-584 and CP1 1189. Alternatively, inhibition of enzymes such as calpain, a calcium-activated proteinase, or caspases (cysteine proteases) may prevent apoptosis.

Protein accumulation appears to be a key feature in the pathogenesis of Parkinson's disease, and agents such as sirolimus (rapamycin), trehalose and small ubiquitin-like modifier (SUMO)-1 appear to prevent protein aggregation. These drugs may be investigated as potential neuroprotective agents.

A new placebo-controlled randomized double-blind multicenter study is under way in the UK to address the safety and efficacy of intermittent bilateral intraputaminal glial cell-line-derived neurotrophic factor (GDNF) infusions administered via convection-enhanced delivery (CED) in people with Parkinson's disease.

Non-motor symptoms. Non-dopaminergic drugs are in development for various non-motor symptoms of Parkinson's disease (Table 9.4).

Gene therapy

Gene delivery is being investigated as a possible treatment for Parkinson's disease, whereby viruses are used as vectors to introduce the DNA of a desired protein into the genome of cells within a specific brain target. It is hoped that this will result in continuous production of the desired therapeutic protein. Most human studies have utilized adeno-associated virus serotype 2 (AAV-2) as the vector, as AAV-2 does not induce an immune response. Three different gene therapy approaches, as outlined below, are currently being tested in Parkinson's disease.

Delivery of the amino acid decarboxylase gene to the striatum to promote the continuous conversion of levodopa to dopamine.

Delivery of the glutamic acid decarboxylase gene (*GAD1*) **to the subthalamic nucleus** (STN) to promote the formation of γ-amino-butyric acid (GABA) to inhibit overactive neuronal firing in the nucleus. An open-label 12-month trial in 12 patients with Parkinson's disease demonstrated significant improvement in Unified Parkinson's Disease Rating Scale (UPDRS) scores with no serious adverse effects.

Gene delivery of neurturin to the striatum. Neurturin is a trophic factor in the glial-cell-line-derived neurotrophic factor (GDNF) family

TABLE 9.4

Treatments under investigation for non-motor symptoms of Parkinson's disease (at the time of publication)

Non-motor symptom	Treatment
Psychosis	• Donepezil
	• Pimavanserin
Depression/anxiety	• Cognitive behavioral therapy
	• Rasagiline
	• Specialist rehabilitation by a MDT
	• Aerobic exercise
Apathy	• Subthalamic deep brain stimulation
	• Amantadine
	• Rivastigmine transdermal patch
Impulse control disorder	• Naltrexone
Sleep/excessive daytime sleepiness	• Naltrexone
	• Rasagiline vs pramipexole
	• Piribedil vs pramipexole or ropinirole
	• Sodium oxybate
Postural hypotension	• Droxidopa
	• Midodrine
	• Pyridostigmine bromide vs fludrocortisone
Hyperactive bladder	• Solifenacin succinate
	• Fesoterodine
Gastrointestinal symptoms	• Rotigotine transdermal patch
	• RM-131 (Relamorelin)
Pain	• Oxycodone/naloxone prolonged release
	• Rotigotine transdermal patch
	• Relaxation guided imagery

MDT, multidisciplinary team.

that has been demonstrated to protect and enhance the function of dopaminergic neurons in both aged and 1-methyl-4-phenyl-1,2,3,6-tetrahydropyridine (MPTP)-lesioned monkeys. In MPTP monkeys, gene delivery resulted in diffuse distribution of GDNF throughout the striatum, which provided motor benefits, restoration of striatal tyrosine hydroxylase (TH) staining and protection of dopaminergic neurons of the substantia nigra zona compacta. Unfortunately, a double-blind study with this agent failed to show superiority over placebo. Further studies are planned to inject neurturin into the nigra, which is the ultimate target for neuroprotection.

Safety of gene therapy is a major concern, as there is the potential of 'off'-medication dyskinesia and tumor formation. It is reassuring, however, that no clinically significant or unanticipated adverse events have been encountered in any of the gene-therapy studies in Parkinson's disease that have been performed to date.

Key references

Gill SS, Patel NK, Hotton GR et al. Direct brain infusion of glial cell derived neurotrophic factor in Parkinson's disease. *Nat Med* 2003;9:589–95.

Jenner P. Treatment of the later stages of Parkinson's disease – pharmacological approaches now and in the future. *Transl Neurodegener* 2015;4:3.

Kieburtz K, Olanow CW. Advances in clinical trials for movement disorders. *Mov Disord* 2015;30:1580–7.

Lang AE, Gill S, Patel NK et al. Randomized controlled trial of intraputamenal glial cell line-derived neurotrophic factor infusion in Parkinson's disease. *Ann Neurol* 2006;59:459–66.

Meltzer HY, Mills R, Revell S et al. Pimavanserin, a serotonin(2A) receptor inverse agonist, for the treatment of Parkinson's disease psychosis. *Neuropsychopharmacology* 2010;35:881–92.

Stocchi F. Therapy for Parkinson's disease: what is in the pipeline? *Neurotherapeutics* 2014;11:24–33.

Tintner R, Jankovic J. Treatment options for Parkinson's disease. *Curr Opin Neurol* 2002;15:467–76.

Useful resources

UK
Association of British
Neurologists
Tel: +44 (0)20 7405 4060
info@abn.org.uk
www.theabn.org

British Association/College of
Occupational Therapists
Tel: +44 (0)20 7357 6480
www.cot.org.uk

Carers UK
Advice Line: 0808 808 7777
Tel: +44 (0)20 7378 4999
info@carersuk.org
www.carersuk.org

The Cure Parkinson's Trust
Tel: +44 (0)20 7487 3892
www.cureparkinsons.org.uk

Disabled Living Foundation
Helpline: 0300 999 0004
Tel: +44 (0)20 7289 6111
info@dlf.org.uk
www.dlf.org.uk

The National Council for
Palliative Care
Tel: +44 (0)20 7697 1520
enquiries@ncpc.org.uk
www.ncpc.org.uk

The Neurological Alliance
Tel: +44 (0)20 7963 3994
arlene.wilkie@neural.org.uk
www.neural.org.uk

Parkinson's Disease Non-Motor
Group
www.pdnmg.com

Parkinson's Disease Nurse
Specialist Association
www.pdnsa.org

Parkinson's UK
Helpline: 0808 800 0303
Tel: +44 (0)20 7931 8080
hello@parkinsons.org.uk
www.parkinsons.org.uk

USA
American Academy of Neurology
Toll-free: 1 800 879 1960
Tel: +1 612 928 6000
www.aan.com

American Association of
Neuroscience Nurses
Toll-free: 1 888 557 2266
Tel: +1 847 375 4733
info@aann.org
www.aann.org

American Parkinson Disease Association
Toll-free: 1 800 223 2732
Tel: +1 718 981 8001
apda@apdaparkinson.org
www.apdaparkinson.org
www.youngparkinsons.org

Caregiver Action Network
Tel: +1 202 454 3970
info@caregiveraction.org
www.caregiveraction.org

LSVT Global
(Lee Silverman Voice Treatment)
Toll-free: 1 888 438 5788
Tel: +1 520 867 8838
info@lsvtglobal.com
www.lsvtglobal.com

The Michael J. Fox Foundation for Parkinson's Research
Toll-free: 1 800 708 7644
www.michaeljfox.org/foundation

National Institute of Neurological Disorders and Stroke
Toll-free: 1 800 352 9424
Tel: +1 301 496 5751
www.ninds.nih.gov

National Parkinson Foundation
Helpline: 1 800 473 4636
contact@parkinson.org
www.parkinson.org

The Parkinson Alliance
Toll-free: 1 800 579 8440
Tel: +1 609 688 0870
www.parkinsonalliance.org

Parkinson's Action Network
Toll-free: 1 800 850 4726
Tel: +1 202 638 4101
info@parkinsonsaction.org
www.parkinsonsaction.org

Parkinson's Disease Foundation
Helpline: 1 800 457 6676
Tel: +1 212 923 4700
info@pdf.org
www.pdf.org

Parkinson's Resource Organization
Toll-free: 1 877 775 4111
Tel: +1 760 773 5628
www.parkinsonsresource.org

International Association of Physiotherapists in Parkinson's Disease Europe
info@appde.eu
www.appde.eu

European Parkinson's Disease Association
info@epda.eu.com
www.epda.eu.com

International Parkinson and
Movement Disorder Society
Tel: +1 414 276 2145
info@movementdisorders.org
www.movementdisorders.org

Parkinson's Association of
Ireland
Toll-free: 1 800 359 359
www.parkinsons.ie

The Parkinson's and Related
Movement Disorders Association
of South Africa
Tel: + 27 (0)11 787 8792
parkinsonassociationsa@gmail.com
www.parkinsons.co.za

Parkinson's Australia
Toll-free: 1 800 644 189
Tel: + 61 (0)407 703 328
info@parkinsons.org.au
www.parkinsons.org.au

Parkinson's New Zealand
Toll-free: 0800 473 4636
Tel: + 64 04 472 2796
info@parkinsons.org.nz
www.parkinsons.org.nz

Parkinson Canada
Toll-free: 1 800 565 3000
Tel: +1 416 227 9700
info@parkinson.ca
www.parkinson.ca

FastTest

You've read the book ... now test yourself with key questions from the authors

- Go to the FastTest for this title
  FREE at fastfacts.com
- Approximate time **10 minutes**
- For best retention of the key issues, try taking the FastTest before and after reading

Index

What the reviewers say

"This book should be on the shelf of every healthcare provider dealing with Parkinson's disease patients." Dr Matthew Stern, Past President, International Parkinson and Movement Disorder Society

"The emphasis on holistic care and improving quality of life for people living with the condition makes this essential reading for the multidisciplinary team." The European Parkinson's Disease Association

"... an invaluable resource for both the novice and more experienced practitioner involved in caring for people living with Parkinson's" Parkinson's Disease Nurse Specialist Association

"... a true success as a didactic source of the latest information in the multidisciplinary care of this condition. It is enriched with comments from people with Parkinson's and spouses, bringing the impact of living with Parkinson's to life. It is an excellent book to consult in a busy practice for all professionals." Mariella Graziano, President, Association of Physiotherapists in Parkinson's Disease Europe, www.appde.eu

"This book is really well done. It is comprehensive and current, yet concise – a must-have for treating PD." David G Standaert MD PhD, Chairman of the Scientific Advisory Committee, American Parkinson Disease Association

"The book is concise and informative, it is easy to navigate and find relevant information quickly. It is a useful resource for both new and experienced healthcare professionals." Louise Ebenezer, Honorary Lecturer, Swansea University; Parkinson's Disease Nurse Specialist, Princess of Wales Hospital

"This [book] does very well in covering a complex area with great clarity and brevity. I would recommend it to anyone studying Parkinson's disease at degree level and it would also be a useful entry level book for those wishing to study it at Masters level." Anthony Duffy MSc BSc(Hons) RN RNT ITEC MBPsS, Senior Lecturer, Swansea University

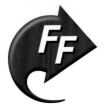

Fast Facts – the ultimate medical handbook series covers over 60 topics, including**:**

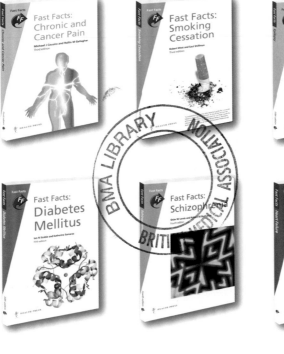

Fast Facts:
Chronic and Cancer Pain
Michael J Cousins and Rollin M Gallagher
Third edition

Fast Facts:
Smoking Cessation
Robert West and Saul Shiffman
Third edition

Fast Facts:
Epilepsy
Martin J Brodie, Steven C Schachter, Patrick Kwan
Revised fifth edition

Fast Facts:
Diabetes Mellitus
Ian N Scobie and Katherine Samaras
Fifth edition

Fast Facts:
Schizophrenia
Shôn W Lewis and Robert W Buchanan
Fourth edition

Fast Facts:
Heart Failure
Dariusz Korczyk, Thomas H Marwick, Gerry Kaye

Fast Facts:
Depression
Mark Haddad & Jane Gunn
Third edition

Fast Facts:
Bladder Disorders
Alex Gleik, Diane K Newman and Alan J Wein
Second edition

Fast Facts:
Multiple Sclerosis
Omar Malik, Ann Donnelly and Michael Barnett
Third edition

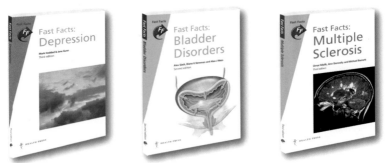

fastfacts.com

Fast Facts

Fast Facts:
Parkinson's Disease

Fourth edition

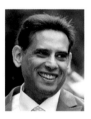

K Ray Chaudhuri MD FRCP DSc
Professor of Neurology and Movement Disorders
Director, National Parkinson Foundation
International Centre of Excellence
King's College London and King's College Hospital
London, UK

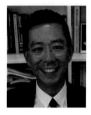

Victor SC Fung MBBS PhD FRACP
Clinical Associate Professor
Sydney Medical School, University of Sydney
Director, Movement Disorders Unit
Department of Neurology, Westmead Hospital
New South Wales, Australia

With additional contribution from Dr Anna Sauerbier,
Clinical Research Fellow, King's College Hospital and King's College,
London, UK.

Declaration of Independence
This book is as balanced and as practical as we can make it.
Ideas for improvement are always welcome: feedback@fastfacts.com

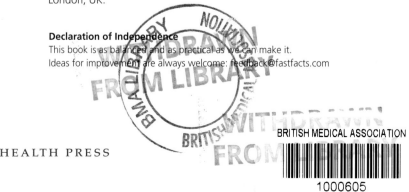

BRITISH MEDICAL ASSOCIATION

1000605

HEALTH PRESS

Fast Facts: Parkinson's Disease
First published 2003; second edition 2007; third edition 2011
Fourth edition May 2016

Text © 2016 K Ray Chaudhuri, Victor SC Fung
© 2016 in this edition Health Press Limited
Health Press Limited, Elizabeth House, Queen Street, Abingdon,
Oxford OX14 3LN, UK
Tel: +44 (0)1235 523233

Book orders can be placed by telephone or via the website.
For regional distributors or to order via the website, please go to:
fastfacts.com
For telephone orders, please call +44 (0)1752 202301 (UK, Europe and Asia–
Pacific), 1 800 247 6553 (USA, toll free) or +1 419 281 1802 (Americas).

Fast Facts is a trademark of Health Press Limited.

A CIP record for this title is available from the British Library.

ISBN 978-1-908541-93-2

Chaudhuri KR (K Ray)
Fast Facts: Parkinson's Disease/
K Ray Chaudhuri, Victor SC Fung

Medical illustrations by Dee McLean, London, and
Annamaria Dutto, Withernsea, UK.
Printed in the UK with Xpedient Print.